Private
Parts

About the Author

Eleanor Thom was born in Sheffield, England. She graduated from Manchester University with a BA in Film and Theatre. On graduation she created the award winning, all female sketch group *Lady Garden* who toured the UK circuit extensively, appearing on TV and Radio and were Edinburgh Fringe Festival favourites. In 2013 she wrote and performed the critically acclaimed character stand-up show *I am Bev*. As an actor she has appeared in *Absolutely Fabulous* (BBC), *Live At The Electric* (BBC) and *Drifters* (Channel 4). Eleanor also writes for other comedians on their live and TV work. This is her first book. She lives in London.

Private Parts

How to really *live* with endometriosis

Eleanor Thom

CORONET

First published in Great Britain in 2019 by Coronet
An Imprint of Hodder & Stoughton
An Hachette UK company

1

A CIP catalogue record for this title is available from the British Library

Hardback ISBN 978 1 473 68755 4
eBook ISBN 978 1 473 68757 8

Typeset in Celeste by Palimpsest Book Production Ltd, Falkirk, Stirlingshire

Printed and bound in Great Britain by Clays Ltd, Elcograf S.p.A.

Hodder & Stoughton policy is to use papers that are natural, renewable
and recyclable products and made from wood grown in sustainable forests.
The logging and manufacturing processes are expected to conform
to the environmental regulations of the country of origin.

Hodder & Stoughton Ltd
Carmelite House
50 Victoria Embankment
London EC4Y 0DZ

www.hodder.co.uk

For my father, Rony Robinson
and
my mother, Viv Thom
without whom I wouldn't be here,
so neither would this book.

Contents

1
Introduction

I am a writer, comedian and woman. I also have endometriosis and I'm sitting in my kitchen with cushions stuffed behind me, a hot-water bottle on my lower back and an overheated wheat bag on my front.

My friend Joe just texted me to say, 'If your illness was a person I'd take it outside and kick it in the dick.' I like this very much, it makes me smile, but I don't visualise the disease as male or female. It's a non-gendered monster, on fire all the time, sometimes great balls of raging fire and sometimes just embers being poked until they raise a little redness. But it's always there, always lit and always threatening to burn down whatever I'm trying to do.

A Crash Course in Endometriosis

Tissue similar to the lining of the uterus (the endometrium) is found in and around the pelvis, attaching to organs and the spaces between them including the uterus, bladder, ovaries, fallopian tubes, uterosacral ligaments and peritoneum (it can also involve other parts like your bowels, intestines, rectum and appendix).

Every month the cells bleed like a period, except in the peritoneal cavity, the blood has nowhere to go and so it stays there, in and among the organs, causing inflammation and pain. Sometimes the disease can stick organs together or form cysts on the ovaries.

Symptoms can include pelvic pain, excessive bleeding, extreme fatigue, nausea and some women experience pain during or after sex. It can cause fertility issues for some women. It may also have an impact on your general physical, mental and emotional well-being. Some women experience these symptoms only during menstruation, but others may experience them more often.

It's not contagious. You can't catch it and you didn't do anything wrong.

Despite evidence to the contrary (I've now written this book) I was fiercely private about my privates and the impact endometriosis had on my life for the best part of twenty years. I didn't tell people about it unless they needed to know. It wasn't because I was embarrassed or because I was trying to make it easier for others not to have an awkward conversation about blood and my genitals. But I didn't want to be judged, victimised or pitied. While I appreciate sympathy, I didn't want endometriosis to define me. I didn't want to *be* the illness. I wanted to be seen as successful and resilient and not struggling with feeble things like 'women's problems'. I also feared people would read the oversimplified headlines and conclude

I had a shit sex life and couldn't have children. I really didn't want my vagina bandied about as gossip, especially if it was going to be incorrect. 'Do you have painful sex?' No, actually. I mean it's painful when they stop talking to you after but that's nothing to do with endometriosis. I've just met some disappointing guys.

I grew up in a staunchly feminist household. Gender was never mentioned in conjunction with achievement or strength so I never viewed being a woman as inferior in any way. However, I was aware of the difficulties women faced in being taken seriously, in being valued and of the misogyny that was knocking around in the big wide world. I was mindful that 'women's problems' could be used against us, to explain our behaviour or dismiss perfectly normal reactions as 'hormonal'. The idea that people might think I was 'hysterical' or exaggerating, and that assumptions would be made about my capabilities, haunted me for a long time and were major reasons why I didn't talk about having endometriosis.

For most of my twenties I worked as a comedian in the all-female sketch act Lady Garden and as a character stand-up. When I first began gigging in 2008 we were often the only women on the bill and despite the rise of some amazing women since, it remains a predominantly male industry. I wanted my work to be taken seriously, I was determined to be seen as equal in terms of being as funny (if not more so) than my male peers, pushing against the mad notion that 'women aren't funny', and that was hard enough already without my misbehaving uterus providing another hindrance. So I kept quiet about it and developed elaborate strategies to manage the symptoms so I didn't miss out on too much or let people down.

Another reason I didn't want to talk about it was that it felt like an insurmountable disease, too complex and never-ending and having to educate people about what it actually *was* each time was exhausting. It also felt futile to discuss it because it wouldn't change anything and inevitably, we'd all just feel depressed. But I want to talk about it now.

I've had endometriosis for twenty-two years and although I have a particularly extreme case, I'm told I'm not a medical marvel. Endometriosis has taken a lot from me but it hasn't taken my ability to laugh, to see the dark comedy in it all. I am a 'peritoneum half-full' kind of gal and this is the book that I looked for but couldn't find when I was lonely, hopeless and in desperate need of a friend who understood what it was like. I wanted something that reflected my experience and recognised the madness of it all, the funny bits and the difficult bits. I wanted something to make it feel less bleak and medical and give me ideas of how to actually *live* with it – that saw me as a person not just a patient. I needed someone to tell me: you're not crazy, you're not imagining it and you're not alone. So this book is the fruit of my loins (literally) and it includes some of the most ridiculous, exasperating and funniest situations I've found myself in with this condition and advice from someone who has lived to tell (and laugh at) the tale. I hope that sharing an honest, intimate account of what it's *really* like to live with this disease will provide some respite, comfort and support for those living with it and give an insight into this secret world and raise awareness for others.

You may find parts of the book very relevant to you and others not so much, because everyone's experience of this disease is different. For me, endometriosis has been destructive, depressing and dramatic, but it's also been pretty funny at times. This won't be everyone's story; some are lucky enough not to be in constant pain, some are less fortunate, some will have a less debilitating version, some might even have it worse. But no one is luckier than the next if they have endometriosis. Whatever your experience, it's likely to have been confusing, upsetting and had an impact on your life.

Endometriosis is persistent but so are we. We can learn skills to live with it, to overcome it. You are not the disease, but it is part of you and working out how to manage it so that it stays a small part and that you have an amazing life despite it is vital.

Because this condition can be inconsistent, I wanted the book itself to reflect this. So you don't have to read it in order, you can flick to the bit you need help with today and ignore my story if it's unhelpful for you. Use it on the days when you need a friend, some advice or a laugh. Use it to help you get through on the good days and the bad, and for the ones where you feel OK, almost.

2
My story

This is not the story I was going to tell

I love stories, you get to live in other people's worlds for a bit; you can dance in the heads of the storytellers for as long as they'll let you. I like stories so much I decided to make my living from them. But when drama happens for real I'm not such a fan, which is funny because I usually love a period drama . . . As a writer you are told to write about what you know, but I didn't want to write about this; I just wanted it to go away so I could get on with making people laugh. But sometimes the story you tell is not the one you thought you were going to. It arrives and plays out whether you like it or not.

Breakfast (age 11½)

We're on holiday in Scarborough, an old-fashioned seaside town in the north of England. Tonight everyone will be here – my mum, sister, cousins, uncles, aunties, grandma – but for now it's just my brother, Dad and me. We came on an early train this morning.

We're in a chintzy cafe on the seafront; the tables are swamped in heavy, starched tablecloths and on top sit plates of overly salted, greasy food, with a hint of salad on the side to show willing. A man near the window smokes a cigarette with one hand while soaking up bean sauce with a slice of white in the other. I've just finished a full English breakfast and I'm already regretting it. I feel nauseous and light-headed. I go to the toilet and find I have bled into my knickers and through to my jeans – ah, that's why I was feeling weird. I've only been having periods for six months and I haven't got the hang of it *at all*. One of the blessings of having a big bottom is that it hides your crotch when you walk, so I'm reassured no one will notice the stain, but I don't have any pads, so I stuff a wodge of toilet paper in my knickers and go back out.

It's the first time I've been away without my mum and because I'm so new to this I don't know what pads to buy or where to get them from. There aren't any supermarkets around here, it's all amusement arcades and candy floss. Back at the table I quietly tell my dad I need to get some stuff. He says we'll keep an eye out for a shop, but he can't think of anywhere either. I'm not totally sure he realises the urgency but I'm glad I have a dad I can talk to, who isn't embarrassed by this. As we leave the cafe my nausea increases, the brisk sea air and the smell of the seafood stall across the road waft over me, and the sick surges up quickly. I panic; the only bin I can see has a lid on top with a narrow mouth and I don't think I can aim that well. I don't make it to the bin. I just throw up on the edge of the road like someone severely hung-over. People stare. My brother goes off to buy me a carton of Ribena to wash away the taste (bottles of water aren't the norm yet). We mount an open-top bus and sit on the top deck, hoping that the breeze and view of the coastline will calm my body. But minutes later I'm holding back the sick again. Frantically trying to work out what to do, I quickly swipe through my options:

a) Lean over the side? An open-top bus is a perfect place to vomit and move on – literally. But it doesn't feel fair to wreck another person's day by hurling on them from above as they walk down the promenade.
b) Focus on deep breaths, try not to be sick at all? The chances of this working are decreasing with every bump on this lumpy coastal road.
c) Swallow any sick that comes up and hope it stays down till I get off at the other end?

TIME'S UP! I vomit purple liquid on to my lap, then on to the floor, trying not to get it on my trainers or the seat or my dad sitting next to me. I can hear my brother making retching noises behind us. I manage to get away with a little on my legs but a lot on my trainers and socks. When we arrive at the other end of the seafront I squelch off the bus embarrassed and shaky. I smell of sick and I just want to lie down but we can't get into the hotel for another five hours. We embark on a slow walk around Peasholm Park, which surrounds a lake with rowing boats and an old organist tinkles away in a glass box that floats in the middle. I feel comforted by the familiarity of this eccentric old-fashioned

English entertainment, but just as I think I might be able to muster through, the organist launches into 'I Do Like to Be Beside The Seaside' and I'm reminded my body doesn't like it much at all. This time I make it to a bin with an open top and just about manage to hold my hair back and avoid being stung by the wasps zizzing around the ice creams melting in the bag below.

* * *

My dad says we *must* get some paracetamol and perhaps something else for me to wear as I'm now wearing more vomit than clothes. Abandoning the park, we walk to town and stumble into one of those everything-you-might need shops: pots and pans next to dressing gowns, huge knickers next to dolls. But for all the everything-you-need-ness of this place, they don't have what *I* need. Instead I get some soft towelling socks and some paracetamol in a bottle, like they have in American films, which makes me feel a bit special and grown up, but still no pads. Although they're not embarrassed by it, my dad and brother have never had to buy them either and none of us thinks to find a phar-macy. Let's hope the toilet roll will hold out. We flag a taxi (a huge treat in the daytime) and when we arrive at the hotel my dad tells the receptionist that 'My daughter is *very* ill and she needs to lie down.' This woman has seen me every summer of my life since I was born. She makes a 'poor you' face and hands us a key, letting us in hours before we're really allowed. I love her. I'm relieved that I can finally lie down but I'm also strangely pleased my dad has said I'm *very* ill; no one has said this or really noticed

9

before. At least my *family* doesn't think I'm exaggerating, that this is normal.

* * *

I don't remember much of the next few hours. My dad draws me a tepid bath and I loll in and out of conscious-ness as the pain contracts. My mother arrives to find me squashed up in a chair in just a t-shirt and my new socks, knees tucked up to my chest. She strokes my head, 'Oh sweetheart. Do you think the greasy food made it worse?' Maybe. She goes out to get some pads, the right ones, the ones I don't know I use.

* * *

Everyone is downstairs in my grandmother's suite having a lovely time and I'm stuck up here. I'm not doing this every month for the rest of my life; you can forget it. I feel ashamed that I'm not resilient like the other women in my family. My grandmother Lily is a strong, stoical woman who has lived through two wars, worked until she was (secretly) seven months pregnant and fought to be allowed to go back to work once she was a mother and a wife. She is funny and laughs a lot, she's clever and well read but she doesn't suffer fools and I feel like I'm letting her down by being weak and 'girly'. I can't tell *her* why I'm ill like this. But I want to see everyone, so I summon the strength to go down. I'm still shaky and I won't have fish and chips like they're having tonight, but at least I'm not still being sick.

And Now . . . Some Myths

Women with endometriosis just have a low pain threshold.
BULLLLSHIT! Women who experience severe and persistent pain actually build up a very high tolerance and incredible psychological skills to keep going in extreme pain, we *rule* with mind over matter.

You must have lots of disease if you're in so much pain.
The severity of the disease and how much pain you're in are *not* connected; some women experience excruciating pain and only have minimal disease, some have advanced disease but very little, or sometimes even no, pain. When the doctors talk about 'superficial' or 'severe' or 'stage 3' it refers to the amount or type of disease *not* how the symptoms are affecting you.

You can't have endometriosis, you're too young.
Symptoms can start from as early as your first period. Severe period pain is not normal. I was told this for years and it delayed diagnosis. Demand further tests, support and a referral to a specialist.

Tampon (age 13)

We're at Center Parcs and I've been in this tiny toilet in our chalet for over an hour, prodding and sweating, trying to get a tampon in. I've had my legs up on the sink, bending forwards, bending backwards, sitting down, squatting, leaning from side to side. It's been like a yoga retreat in here.

My dad has taken my brother and sister to the swimming pool and my mum is waiting impatiently in the kitchen for me to 'Just put it in and let's go!' But it's not that easy. I can't get this bastard thing *in* – I can't get the angle right. All the other women who have periods don't seem to have this problem; the adverts look like they just pop it in and go about their day. Maybe I'm not built to fit tampons? I'm so tired, so sore, it feels like someone has punched me in the ass, like someone is pummelling my uterus and this swirling pain in my back doesn't show signs of stopping. Can't I just stay here and sleep?

MY MUM: *You do everything you always do.*
My mum is a feminist and, as such, she is fiercely against anything that is designed to slow you down or hinder you as a woman.

MY MUM: *It's not like years ago when women took to their beds.*
Sounds ideal to me, I'd love to take to my bed, or anyone's bed, frankly, just let me lie down on the floor here and quietly pass out and I'll be grateful.

My story

MY MUM: *You don't want to wear pads every month for the rest of your life, it's like wearing nappies!*
It's not like I haven't *tried* to use tampons before now, after all I have been bleeding for two years and it isn't exactly light. Tampons would be much easier, more invisible, less faffy and probably more absorbent. But I have already spent a great deal of time grappling with them, trying to get them to go in and stay in without feeling like a piece of cardboard is digging at my insides – they're so uncomfortable. I couldn't crack it, so I just gave up.

MY MUM: *We swim, we run, we work. You don't stop doing things just because you're menstruating. It's perfectly normal and natural. Women don't stop for this.*
It irks me, her determination to use the proper words. 'Menstruating' makes it sound like something from an old textbook, so clinical and detached. I want to say that this doesn't feel like anything I've ever read about, it doesn't *feel* normal. It feels like someone is using my uterus as a bouncy castle and launching themselves off the walls. There's so much blood too, like a bottle is tipped upside down and it's pouring out of me.

MY MUM: *All the women I know use tampons, they'd never dream of using towels.*
I keep fiddling. My right leg is now somehow miraculously up on the cistern. I'm bending over but I can't see the entrance – how do you do it blind? How do other women do it? Shouldn't there be a class for this? The leaflet with squiggly sketches of a woman doing it is entirely useless. Although there is little detail in the drawings, the implicit suggestion is

that she's finding it really easy. I bet she's got the luxury of inserting hers in a bigger room. I bet she's not thirteen years old and I bet she's not got her mum hurrying her on the other side of the door. I stuff the leaflet back in the box, it's not helping, it just reminds me I'm no good at this.

MY MUM: We do everything we do for the other twenty-one days of the month. You're not dying. It's perfectly natural. It *feels* like I'm dying! I want to scream. I'm pale, weak and nauseous. Everything already felt swollen and now it's throbbing too because I'm aggravating it. I was so looking forward to being a grown-up, but I've fallen at the first hurdle, I'm failing miserably. I can't do it, let me go back to being a girl again.

Finally I think I've managed it, but it's not very comfortable. My mum is relieved that it's done, unaware that this has been quite a distressing experience. Once we get to the pool, I'm very anxious that it's going to come out, unbeknown to me, and I will only notice it when I, and everyone else, see it bobbing in the water behind me. It doesn't fall out of course. I have yet to learn that you *know* if a tampon has moved. Rather annoyingly, my mum is right- it *is* freeing and I get a strange sense of belonging, that I'm part of this secret club of women; I am swimming *and* menstruating but no one knows, my period hasn't stopped me. As the teenage boys nudge and smile I realise an upside to being a grown-up is my rather large breasts, so that's something to be happy about I suppose.

* * *

My story

The bit in between (age 11–17)

I didn't keep diaries or pay attention to my cycle. Not being informed was a coping strategy. If I knew when it was coming I would be counting down the days, too conscious of this looming ghastly experience. It felt like the best way to stop it taking over my life. It meant I didn't pre-empt it and say no to stuff or move things around it, and it helped me to avoid extra anxiety about whether it would come on the day of an exam or a party. My logic was that I'd just deal with it if it happened, which gave me a sense of control when there actually wasn't any. It seemed to make sense at the time, but it often meant I had to leave things urgently, throw away a lot of knickers and I went thought an extraordinary amount of Vanish. This strategy led to a development of an unhealthy relationship with the symptoms; my reaction to their sudden onset was panicked and urgent- 'fighting', and I know now that this response puts further stress on your body which may make the pain worse.

THINGS I KNOW NOW

- Keeping track of your cycle can give you *more* control over your mood, pain and other symptoms.

- Period tracker apps such as *Clue*, *Flo* and *Eve* help you to monitor your cycle and symptoms, which means you can prepare better. Although understanding *why* the symptoms are happening at certain times doesn't stop them happening, it does help you to make sense of it and to know it will pass.

• Situations of heightened stress and pressure e.g. exams or big work events can exacerbate symptoms, so if you then have to handle something unpredictable such as your period starting that day it will make everything worse – it sometimes helps to know so you can prepare.

Good morning, good morning (age 16)

Waking up in sheets of cold, yet sort of warm, sticky blood is unnerving. I haven't ever seen blood like this in real life, bright red with some darker clots and *so* much of it. My bed looks like that scene in *The Godfather,* but where the horse's head should be is me, in a tight foetal position desperately hoping I can just go back to sleep and not have to deal with this. My parents have just split up and my mum has moved out, my grandfather is dying and my GCSEs are in a few weeks. Great timing uterus, thanks.

It feels like the middle of the night but it can't be, it's getting light outside. I use all my fight to get to the bathroom and lie on the cold, hard floor, which is delightfully soothing. Opening a window would help but the idea of moving again seems impossible. If I just lie really still perhaps it will go, maybe it will die down or jump out of my body, escaping like a demon. I get very short waves of relief but not enough to recoup before the next contraction and surge of nausea. Something feels really wrong and I'm not in control of this.

On hands and knees I make my way to the cupboard and rake through the medicine drawer. It's full of empty packets for Oraldene and Bonjela, old bottles of ancient, long-gone syrups and capsules for indigestion, but no painkillers. I'm desperate. I'll take anything, I don't care, but I don't know what will work. What if I take something I'm not supposed to and it makes me even sicker? I can't risk that. I crawl back to the toilet.

This pain is much worse than it has ever been. Surely I've lost like eight pints of blood now? Maybe I'm dying. Maybe something has burst inside. My mind is rushing and I'm panicking, but I'm also too exhausted to panic. I want my mum but she isn't here. I look at the clock, 5 a.m. When is an OK time to wake someone up because you have bad periods? This can't be what all women go through every month because everyone would be talking about it, wouldn't they? For the next few hours I pass out and sleep between bouts of vomiting and diarrhoea, and when it's a reasonable time, I wake my dad. I don't know what's going on but I can't do this on my own any more.

* * *

We go to A&E. The receptionist demands that *I* explain my symptoms and not my dad or sister, after all I am sixteen now, not a child. Her tone suggests that if it's bad enough I'll ask for help but if I can't even summon the strength to fight for myself then it can't be *that* bad. But this doesn't make sense, if it's really bad I wouldn't be able to speak at all would I? We wait for hours on the hard plastic chairs with no pain relief, I sporadically vomit into a cardboard bowl and slump on my sister as she strokes my hair. Eventually I see a doctor, who presses my tummy and rules out appendicitis. His incredulity and impatience is clear: why are you making such a fuss about something as routine as periods? Perhaps it's food poisoning, or IBS, either way we can't help, see your GP if you're still suffering in a few days. But my mum took me to the GP years ago and he just told me it was bad periods – sorry – won't he just say that again? I am told to go home, take some paracetamol and try to sleep; hopefully it will settle down. I hope next month won't be like this. I can't miss my exams.

3
Getting a diagnosis

Why is early diagnosis important?

If you get the right help early enough, not only does it reduce unnecessary pain, stress and suffering, but it can also limit the growth of the disease. If endometriosis has been left unmanaged for a long time, treatment can be more difficult and less effective and you may require surgery rather than more conservative ways to manage the symptoms (such as hormone treatments).

THINGS I KNOW NOW

- Getting the right diagnosis can be life-changing; many women find their symptoms are hugely alleviated by hormone or surgical treatments.

- If everyone knows what it actually *is* it can be managed much better, by doctors and by women themselves.

- Don't suffer in silence and don't be deterred by misdiagnoses, keep asking for the right help until you get it.

It's not endometriosis, it must be . . .

A major reason for the delay in diagnosis is that endometriosis is a complex disease with a myriad of symptoms that can be confused with other conditions. It's also made more difficult because symptoms vary for each woman and they may not be constant, cyclical or 'textbook' endometriosis. Many women are repeatedly told their symptoms are either normal or they are misdiagnosed with something else: appendicitis, IBS, UTIs, pelvic inflammatory disease, sometimes even a mental-health issue. For years I'd been struggling with bowel issues, vomiting, passing out, regular urinary infections, but I didn't know that these were all major symptoms of a disease I had never heard of. I thought I'd look like a hypochondriac saying, 'Oh and by the way, here are a load of other things I have too.' I didn't realise they were all connected so I didn't think to mention them, and doctors didn't ask. This is where lack of awareness has serious consequences: if *doctors* don't know much about it either, then they won't know what to look for and women will continue to go undiagnosed.

Getting a diagnosis

Midnight feast (age 17)

There is a woman lying in the bed next to me eating the best part of a family pack of Quavers and telling me about her prolapsed bladder. She is nil-by-mouth, which means she shouldn't be eating anything because she is having surgery first thing tomorrow, but she assures me that 'these are basically just air so I think it's fine'. I am in a gynaecology ward with three other women: one is recovering from a miscarriage, one has just had a hysterectomy and the other is my prolapsed friend. Our private parts jumbled together in one ward, lots of 'women's problems' in here. The other women are kind, but they are much older than me, facing life-changing situations. I'm not one of them, I just have bad periods, don't I? I want to be eating ice cream in bed with my new boyfriend and dancing at nightclubs with my friends, I don't want to be listening to stories about dangling bits and how we should 'use it or lose it'. It's like being in a gynaecological version of *A Christmas Carol*; the ghost of female future is warning me about what might come. Being confronted with how our bodies can betray and humiliate us, how they can get so out of control, is terrifying.

This is my first real experience of hospitals. Apart from one trip to the GP when I was twelve and A&E a year earlier, I hadn't sought any further help. But I collapsed at school yesterday so they brought me in. Doctors, medical students, specialists – everyone has seen me. I've had all the scans, exams and blood tests they can offer but no one can work out what's wrong. I've just started the contraceptive pill and part of me is worried all of this is my fault. I've been dating my boyfriend for six months and started being sexually active (and by God we were being active) for the first time. I should have known my body would have something to say about all this fun. Perhaps this was my fault, not for having sex, but for messing about with my delicate system, by putting these alien hormones in my body?

* * *

It's also the first time I've had hospital food and it's not great, guys. Bland, beige and somehow it all tastes the same. Oh and *everything* comes with sweetcorn. You're asked to choose your *dinner* while you're eating your *breakfast*, which is served at 8 a.m. prompt, an impossible hour for digestion when you have been up for most of the night in pain. Then before you've even finished your porridge or muesli or what-ever it is you can't remember you ordered and now can't distinguish with eye or tongue, someone turns up demanding you get out of bed and suggests a bath! It's not much fun being on other people's timetables when you're this poorly.

* * *

Although this ward is full of women, is run by women and is focused on 'women's problems', there isn't as much empathy as you might expect. There is a 'get up and out' attitude displayed by the staff. Every evening they encourage us to eat in the day room: a drab, draughty space at the end of the ward, with a hodgepodge collection of chairs and a long table. It will do us good to get out of bed. I know they're right, but it feels a bit much when everyone is feeling so weak and sick. As we sit there in our dressing gowns with greasy hair and pale faces, IV wires dangling from our arms, I'm struck by the solidarity in the room. All of us sitting here with our bits buggering us about, saying how we daren't laugh too much in case we wee or it all falls out. There is fortitude in women when we are pushed to our limit, especially when we're in it together. Somehow we find strength and compassion for others in a way that moves me to tears. I am reminded that women are pretty amazing in a crisis, that they still find a way to smile and laugh, so at least I'm here with them.

* * *

Family, friends and my boyfriend come to visit, my dad makes up stories and my mum brushes my hair and pushes for answers. I wish they could stay but visitors are only allowed to be here for a couple of hours a day. Occasionally the kinder nurses let them stay a little longer and one night, well after visiting is over, my mum (against all her better judgement) sneaks in a McDonald's to cheer me up. I shuffle to the empty day room and wolf down a lukewarm burger and fries by the light of the moon. Sometimes a little bit of what you fancy does you good (even when it isn't technically good for you) and sometimes the little things make the difficult things less difficult. Eventually, unable to determine the reason I feel so ill, they say I can go home to rest instead, so I do. Still undiagnosed.

What Happens in an Internal Exam?

You might feel nervous because you don't know what will happen – try not to worry, it's over quickly and doctors and nurses do them all the time so there's no need to be embarrassed.

- You lie on a bed with your feet in stirrups and your legs apart, or maybe lie flat with your feet together and knees flopped out to each side, so your legs are apart in a kind of diamond shape.
- The doctor will wear vinyl gloves and use lubricant jelly to make it less uncomfortable for your when they insert their finger into your vagina.
- They may use a speculum, a contraption they insert into your vagina that gently widens it so that they can see better – also used during cervical smear tests.
- They may press gently on the walls of your vagina using a finger, asking whether there is any pain or discomfort. They may also take some swabs and this might sting for a moment.

Tips
- Somehow, no matter how much you wipe, there is an infinite amount of lubricant jelly left on you after the exam, so wear a nice pair of full cotton knickers. (I learnt this the hard way – I wore a thong the first time.)
- Keep breathing. Your instinct will be to clench and hold your breath if you are nervous or it's uncomfortable.

Paradoxically, this protective reflex will actually make it worse. Try to relax and think of something nicer to distract you – a cherished memory, a favourite holiday destination or something coming up that you're looking forward to. This is a useful thing to be able to do for any procedure – blood tests, scans, examinations.

What Happens in an Ultrasound Scan?

- An external ultrasound scan is like the one they use for seeing babies. The sonographer/radiologist will squeeze some jelly on your abdomen (it's a bit chilly) and press an ultrasound wand around. It might be a little uncomfortable if you have bloating or it's a particular time in your cycle.
- They might also do a transvaginal scan (sometimes called an 'internal scan') to get a clearer picture of your reproductive organs. They insert a thin ultrasound probe into your vagina and move it around gently to look for disease and cysts. Sometimes disease can be seen and diagnosed this way rather than through surgery.
- BUT this is not a definitive diagnostic test; you may still have disease that can't be seen on a scan (I did, and do, have spots of disease that can't be seen this way). Being able to see disease also depends on the skill and experience of the sonographer.

Tips

- A sonographer is an expert in ultrasound, but they might not be experienced in endometriosis; being able to see disease on a scan is still a skill that is highly specialised. It's likely your consultant will read the scan report afterwards and determine the next stage of treatment.
- They might be quiet while they take the images; don't panic, it doesn't necessarily mean bad news, they're just concentrating.
- Ask to look. I used to be too freaked out to do this, preferring to stare at the ceiling until it was done, but now I ask them to turn the screen and explain to me what they're seeing. Understanding it helps to calm me down.
- Take some paracetamol or ibuprofen before. Internal examinations can be uncomfortable if you have endometriosis.
- Remember that breathing thing? It helps here too.

What Happens After These Investigations?

You might have to wait to see your doctor to discuss any findings, which can be frustrating and worrying. You also might also feel a bit sore and emotional. I recommend you take yourself off and do something cheerful: treat yourself to a little something, a cake and a warm drink, talk to a friend or someone you love. Doing something enjoyable after these appointments gives you some control back.

Number One (age 17)

The good thing about having been in hospital is that once you're in the system they have to follow up. Six months later, via a colorectal surgeon who considered exploratory surgery for Crohn's disease (err, no thanks, I don't think that's what this is), I'm back in gynae outpatients. A wonderful female registrar asks questions and apologises for having to do *another* internal exam, but by this point I don't care, I just want to know what's wrong. She's concerned about pain in particular areas, as coupled with the symptoms it matches her working diagnosis. I think the word endometriosis gets mentioned, but it's a bit fuzzy because I'm overwhelmed by her skill and consideration. She is the first doctor to really *listen*. Instead of taking a coffee break that day she spent a little longer with me and for that, I am eternally grateful. I'm not sure what would have happened next if she hadn't. She books me in for exploratory surgery with her consultant, Dr B.

* * *

Three months later a kind male nurse helps me into a preheated bed and I make some quip about how wonderful the NHS is – that it's like being in a hotel. I haven't quite worked out how to be a patient yet, so I revert back to what I do in any situation that feels a bit uneasy and make light of it all. But I don't feel very light – this suddenly feels quite serious. Lots of people bustle around me putting in needles and taking my blood pressure. The nurse places a pillow under my knees and explains that it helps with abdominal pain because it stops the muscles being stretched (a trick I use to this day). I'm wheeled into the little holding room where the anaesthetist talks casually like he's knocking up a sandwich rather than a potion that will knock me out, but his matter-of-fact manner is reassuring, this is obviously routine, nothing to worry about. He puts a cannula needle into the back of my hand and asks me to count down from a hundred. I panic, my fear of maths kicks in – what if I can't do it? I'm going to look stupid – 100, 99, 98. . .

And then I'm in recovery, floating in and out of consciousness. A loud Yorkshire woman is slapping my hand and shouting:

NURSE: Hello, Eleanor? Eleanor love, can you hear me? Something must be wrong, no one ever uses my full name unless I'm in trouble. I can't speak – oh my God I can't speak, what's happened? I realise an oxygen mask is covering my mouth. I try to instruct my head to nod.

NURSE: Eleanor sweetheart, how's the pain? If you could number it, ten being the highest, one the lowest, what would you say your pain is?
Because I'm in and out of consciousness the pain hasn't registered yet but as she says the word everything suddenly feels very swollen and sore. My mouth is dry, I murmur through the mask – eight. She squeezes the morphine into my hand, but the sensation is weird, it starts from my feet up to my head, like I'm a bottle being filled up. Morphine is not quite as pleasurable as you are led to believe, your body sort of resists it, your muscles become rigid and push against it, like your veins are already full and there's no room for this

28

thank you! Then there's the nausea and you feel like you're on the cusp of fainting, and then – only then – is it amazing, the pain is gone.

* * *

Dr B hovers above me looking down, everything is blurry, white and bright, like when they show heaven in films. He's trying to tell me what he's found, but I can't make sense of anything, of course I can't, I'm smacked off my head. I squeeze his hand in an attempt to say thank you. He smiles and drifts off and so do I.

When I wake up I'm back on the ward with my mum sitting next to me. I'm drowsy and not quite sure where I am. Dr B arrives.

DR B: So we looked inside and you have quite a lot of endo-metriosis. We haven't done anything today but we need to see you for another surgery to remove it in a couple of months. You have a lot of disease for your age; I think it's been growing for quite some time. Let's focus on the next surgery and then look at hormonal ways to manage it.
My brain gets very busy. I don't know anything about this or anyone with it, it's just periods isn't it? You can fix *that* can't you? How have I got this? Did I do something wrong? Why didn't anyone notice earlier? I have my A-level exams in a couple of months, I don't have time for illness and opera-tions, could it be anything else? But this is also the moment I stop thinking about periods as periods; they are now a disease, they're not natural or normal, they're painful because something is *wrong*.

* * *

It's the middle of the night and I'm back at home sitting on the toilet in a woozy state. My tummy is hard and distended, so much so that I can't see my bits underneath. I think that this is what it will be like when I'm older and pregnant. I can't decipher whether I need a wee or it's just pressure and bruising in my abdomen. My head is dizzy with thoughts and fears about what this diagnosis might mean; my brain feels swollen too. I notice a rusty-orange substance, like fake tan, smeared across my tummy and going down on to my thighs. What is this? It reminds me of that stuff we used in a science experiment once, and then I think of the strange teachers we had, which is not a thought you want to have when you don't have your knickers on. Your brain makes funny cognitive leaps when you're coming down from the anaesthetic and morphine: things leap up, connect, break up and sort of fit together confused and disjointed. Back in bed as I drift off, I remember – it's iodine of course. A week later I go to my eighteenth birthday party and dance cautiously but joyfully. Three months later I have excision surgery and a month after that, despite some residual discomfort, I sit my exams.

What Really Happens When You Have Surgery?

- A laparoscopy is keyhole surgery. It usually involves a little cut in or just under your belly button and a few little cuts at the top of your pubic hair line or lower abdomen.

- It's usually an outpatient procedure so you're in and out within the day. But you might stay overnight if the surgery is longer than anticipated or your pain levels feel unmanageable.
- Before you go down, they ask you to change into a gown and some paper knickers (they are weird; like a shower cap with leg holes).
- The consultant and anaesthetist usually come to see you before to explain the risks and you sign a consent form. Don't be afraid to ask questions or discuss any worries at this point.
- You'll be taken down to the surgery ward where they will give you a general anaesthetic. Then you're unconscious and they take you into theatre.
- In the operation they inflate your abdomen with carbon dioxide gas so they can see everything clearly. Although they push out as much of the gas as possible, it can take a few days for it to go down.
- Don't panic if you feel a bit 'blown up' afterwards. The gas might travel around your body as it disperses; sometimes you can even feel discomfort in your shoulders. Moving around (even slowly) helps it go quicker post-op.
- When you wake up, you'll probably feel woozy, nauseous and sore.
- If you are in a lot of pain in the recovery room *take the meds!* It's unlikely they will give you morphine or very strong medication again after this point.

What About the Recovery Time?

- If it is exploratory surgery (assessing the disease without removing it) the recovery time can be anything from a few days to a couple of weeks.
- If they laser or excise the disease, recovery can be longer. It will depend on how much they have done and your own levels of pain and discomfort.
- Although it appears (from the outside) to be a minor operation, it *is* major surgery if they have tried to remove the disease.
- You need to be patient and give yourself time to recover.
- You might feel groggy from the general anaesthetic, but don't worry, it fades.
- The more operations I have had, the longer the recovery has taken each time. The operation may aggravate pre-existing scar tissue and inflammation.
- It's important to take the pain medication your doctor has suggested; your body needs respite from the pain in order to recoup and heal.

THINGS I KNOW NOW

- Be cautious of doctors who diagnose or operate too quickly just because they've hit a dead end in their investigations.

- Getting the wrong diagnosis or treatment delays the help you really need. You might need to be strong and push for this – you *know* your body. Remember when they thought it might be my intestines? I knew it wasn't that, so said no to an exploratory surgery.

Talking to myself

ME 17: So what is it again?

ME NOW: En-doe-me-tree-oh-sis.

ME 17: Never heard of it, it must be rare then?

ME NOW: No, actually, it's the second most common gynae condition and statistics suggest it affects 1 in 10 women – that's 1.6 million women in the UK and 7 million in the US. So you've definitely met someone with it.

ME 17: But they know how to fix it yeah?

ME NOW: Not so much, it's more about managing it, but there's lots of stuff you can try and you don't have to suffer on your own any more, that's the good news.

ME 17: Why don't they know how to fix it, is it a 'new' thing?

ME NOW: Tell me about it. No, the earliest case was in 1860 . . .

ME 17: Christ! The doctor didn't really explain it so I just looked it up. It's weird reading about something you've been experiencing for years thinking it was normal.

ME NOW: I know, I'm sorry you didn't know earlier. You're going to get help now, it gets easier, sort of.

ME 17: That sounds ominous . . . Any other advice?

ME NOW: Yeah, keep reading.

10 Things You Need to Know About Endometriosis

1. **Endometriosis is different for everyone**: symptoms, disease, efficacy of treatments and their side effects are different for each woman.

2. **Currently there is no cure**: but there may be better symptom suppressors that you haven't tried yet. Finding the best treatment for you might be a bit of trial and error; it's about getting a balance between managing symptoms and the effects. You might also need to change treatments over time based on your symptoms and life plans.

3. **Find an endometriosis specialist**: it's important to see someone who fully understands the disease; what to look for and how to treat and manage it. You may need to push for this. You can find your nearest endometriosis centre in the UK at the BSGE (British Society for Gynaecological Endoscopy) website (see page 341) or ask your doctor for a referral to a specialist.

4. **Beware of medical terms**: when doctors say 'minimal' or 'superficial' or refer to 'stages' of disease, it can feel like they are diminishing your symptoms. They aren't, these are medical terms for the type of disease, referring to the location, size and depth of the endometrial deposits. Remember that the amount of disease does not correlate to how much pain you're in, and vice versa.

5. **Surgery isn't always the answer**: it's not a quick fix and it doesn't cure the disease. Depending on your case it may be that the disease can be suppressed and managed

with medication and hormone therapy rather than surgery. Talk to your doctor about what they think is the best plan for *you*.

6. **It is a long-term condition but don't be too despairing yet**: it doesn't automatically mean you will be in pain all the time, that the symptoms can't be managed or that it will *definitely* affect your fertility. Try not to assume that the versions you read about online, in medical textbooks or even my version in this book is going to be *your* experience. Not every symptom, treatment or setback will automatically happen to you. Hopefully you won't need much intervention, and if you do it won't be forever. You might have bad patches and harder times but mostly you will be OK (if a little more tired than you used to be).

7. **Try not to assume the worst**: it doesn't necessarily progress or get worse over time for *everyone*. A diagnosis doesn't mean you're going to be ill forever or that it won't get better or become easier to manage. Many women live very full lives with endometriosis, even if they undergo hormonal treatments or surgery at various points. There is a lot of hope out there. Focus on finding the best possible treatment (or combination of treatments) for *you*.

8. **You might be in denial**: you might rail against the diagnosis for a bit (I know I did), want to ignore it, determined that it won't change your life. It's a totally natural response to the diagnosis of a long-term health problem. Let it be, it's part of processing, take your time, you'll know when you need to address it or get more support.

9. **You're not on your own**: there are 200 million women who have it (to varying degrees) all around the world. You might want to access online support, go to a group and talk to fellow sufferers for advice.

10. **But it's OK to want to be on your own**: if you don't want to be part of a group, or you'd rather not talk about it, that's OK (I did this for fifteen years). But in the darkest of hours know that others are going through it too; you will get through this and it will get easier. Reach out for help, even if it's just to doctors or close friends and family.

It only took seven years then!

I had been developing endometriosis from the age of eleven with no diagnosis, treatment or support. It had been spreading like black treacle in and around my organs, stretching and pulling them together. No wonder I was passing out every month! Doctors had told me this was nothing to worry about, so I just got used to the symptoms that were increasing and worsening over the years. It took seven years for someone to take this seriously and recognise the life-disrupting monthly symptoms. The delay in my diagnosis was directly connected to the lack of awareness of the condition in both society and within medicine. I was let down by the health system but also by my *own* ignorance of this condition. I didn't tell them the right information and they didn't ask the right questions.

It was *chance* that I collapsed at school and my friend took me to hospital. Had I been alone at home I would have continued to think not much of it. It was *chance* that I saw that doctor who led me to Dr B, who was by *chance* an endometriosis specialist. I want to think this 'chance diagnosis' couldn't happen to another young woman today. That she wouldn't be fobbed off quite so easily, for quite so long, but I fear there is still so much ignorance and misunderstanding around this condition and without better awareness women and doctors won't even know what signs to look for. This must change.

Being undiagnosed and dismissed for years can have a huge impact on mental health. Many women botch their way through, trying to manage the condition on their own and hoping it will get better. Statistics suggest that it takes an average of seven to ten years to get a diagnosis. If your GP's knowledge of endometriosis is limited, they may be missing key signifiers that would speed up referral, diagnosis and a better treatment plan. The chances of being dismissed or misdiagnosed are increased if you are very young or do not mention that your symptoms are related to your periods.

Ask if there is a GP who specialises in women's health, they might have a better understanding of endometriosis and the clinical pathways that lead you to a specialist.

Things to think about before a GP appointment

It's hard to remember everything in the moment but your symptoms may be very significant. Make some notes ahead of seeing your doctor.

- Keep a diary of your cycle, symptoms and pain levels.
- When are the symptoms or pain worse?
- Is there any change at certain times in your cycle?

- Do you have multiple symptoms at once?
- Do you use any birth control? Has this changed recently?
- Have you changed anything in your lifestyle that might be useful for the doctor to know (e.g. diet/job)?
- Has it got any worse or better over time? Can *you* link that to anything?
- What aggravates your symptoms and pain? (E.g. sex, bowel movements, sleep, ovulation.)
- Keep a food diary; they're going to ask you to do this anyway if they think it's IBS or vitamin deficiencies.

I know this is a ball-ache (uterus-ache?) and you have much more joyous things to be doing with your time, but by charting your symptoms you have evidence of what is happening each month and that is hard for a doctor to ignore. It can also give you a sense of control and it's the best thing *you* can do to ensure better treatment and help. You won't regret it.

Why do I need a specialist?

If your GP or gynaecologist has limited understanding or experience of endometriosis you might find yourself on the wrong treatments, being operated on unnecessarily and not being listened to. Endometriosis surgery is also complex, so if the surgeon is not familiar with the disease they may not know how to operate on it efficiently, or the surgery may be too intricate. This can potentially leave endometrial deposits untreated, which can mean little change to symptoms and maybe even more surgery in the future. At worst, ignorance could result in more drastic surgery and because there are many nerves and sophisticated interconnected systems in the pelvic region, the ramifications of getting it wrong can be great.

I spoke to Davor Jurkovic, consultant gynaecologist and the director of Gynaecology Diagnostic and Outpatient Treatment at University College Hospital, London:

As long as you have an accurate pre-operative diagnosis, surgery for endometriosis can be carried out safely and effectively. However if a general gynaecologist finds the disease acciden-tally, they would be compelled to do something. Although they may be well trained in general pelvic surgery, they would not be able to tackle *severe* disease. They may be able to deal with the so-called 'mild' or 'moderate' disease but they are not going to appreciate how serious the disease is because they will not look in the space in the pelvis where other disease may be. If the surgery for severe endometriosis is done, it should be done by a dedicated specialist not by a casual surgeon.

A referral to an endometriosis specialist is not automatic, you may need to ask. Your pathway to see one is reliant on your GP's knowl-edge of who to refer you to. If they don't know of a specialist you'll likely be referred to a general gynaecologist in the first instance. Also, there may not be a specialist at your local hospital, but you can ask your doctor to find the nearest one. If you are meeting with a general gynaecologist initially, ask about their experience with the disease, and if you don't feel reassured, ask if you can see a specialist. Having an endometriosis specialist has been vital for me; it's helped me feel less fearful, lonely and confused.

At the Endo-the Day

I think we should be given one hour with a specialist endo-metriosis nurse or doctor when we're first diagnosed to:

- fully understand our individual disease, possible treatment options and prognosis.
- ask questions about pain, symptom management and fertility.

It would lessen confusion and myths and empower us to work with doctors as a team. I *know* that knowledge helps reduce years of anxiety, stress, wasted trips to hospital and unnecessary tests. One hour to change a lifetime. Not much is it?

Things can only get better

In 2017, the National Institute for Health and Care Excellence (NICE) published new guidelines in an attempt to reduce the gap between symptoms and diagnosis. The report said:

Healthcare professionals need to:
- be more aware and alert to the symptoms.
- listen better to the patient's concerns and refer them to a gynaecologist and/or endometriosis specialist if they are reporting persistent symptoms including pelvic pain, severe period pain, pain during sex and fertility issues.
- refer women with confirmed deep-seated disease to a specialist endometriosis doctor or centre.

- not rule out endometriosis:
  - even if the patient is 17 and under.
  - even if the patient continues to have symptoms after tests or initial examinations come back clear (such as ultrasounds).

The medical system should provide:
- gynaecology departments with doctors who specialise in endo-metriosis.
- a managed network of care including GPs, nurses, sexual-health clinics who should be conscious and alert to the symptoms.

These guidelines are a significant step forwards, especially because they highlight the importance of being referred to a specialist and the need for wider awareness and understanding of endometriosis across the health system. While doctors will have an understanding of this disease, they are not always *experts* in endometriosis, and this can be a problem, particularly for women who have more complex, rather than 'textbook' disease. Because so little is known about endometriosis, it's important that the doctor treating you has a thorough understanding of what we *do* know and that they tailor the treatment to suit *your* disease and plans.

Can they fix it then?

I assumed (naively) that now they knew what it was, it could be fixed, I would have an operation and move on. I didn't need to be educated about it. Because of this I didn't do much research. I half-read the leaflet the doctor gave me and looked it up in my grandmother's ancient encyclopaedia which spelt it 'endometritus', which sounded too much like detritus and that felt a bit unpleasant so I stopped reading. I saw something about it being 'a career woman's' disease but that sounded pretty sexist and it couldn't be true anyway, I hadn't even *started* my career yet, surely this wasn't punishment for working hard at school?

In my defence, there wasn't much information to find back then either. In 2002 the Internet was only just emerging, so searching for information on Google, patient forums or charity websites wasn't possible yet. All I could find were medical books and they just made me depressed. So I decided to think of it as something I had but it wasn't going to change anything. But from the age of seventeen my life stopped and started. Roughly every eighteen months, just as I'd managed to claw back my abdominal muscles and start my life back up again, I had to have another surgery. My current tally is nine (I'm hoping to get the tenth for free; like a coffee loyalty card).

Dr B's Marvellous Medicine

Dr B was honest and thorough when I was diagnosed, but he didn't panic me about endometriosis or my prognosis. Crucially, he didn't let on how bad mine would become. This was extremely kind on his part. If he had, I might have made life decisions based on disease, not dreams and I would have missed out on some amazing things. Instead, he kept a close and vigilant eye on me. I am very lucky; many people do not have this. I am also very grateful to him for making the scars so small I can still wear a bikini.

Some More Myths

You've got it because you delayed having children/put your career first.
Endometriosis is not caused by any decisions you have made. It's not punishment or because of anything, it's bad luck. Some women may find a genetic link, but many women don't have anyone in their family with it. There is nothing you could have done differently, just concentrate on getting the right support *now*.

Having a baby is a cure.
Some women may get respite from symptoms during the pregnancy, but find they return afterwards. The change of hormones can be a suppressive treatment, not curative.

Endometriosis means you can't have children.
Age has the biggest impact on fertility, as with *every* woman, but whether endometriosis affects your fertility will depend on where your disease is and how long it has been left untreated. Infertility is not an inevitable symptom for *all* women with endometriosis. *Please* speak to your doctor if you're worried about this (more on this later, see page 229).

What do I do now?

It's a lot to take in when you're first diagnosed. You may have a lot of fear, confusion and worry about short-term and very long-term things, playing out all the possible scenarios in your head, wondering what this might mean for you and the rest of your life. Emotions can be contradictory and complex and they can all exist at once. Be patient with yourself, you need time to come to terms with it and what adjustments you might need to make around it. It's also important to recognise that if you have been dealing with symptoms for years without being heard, it might feel anti-climactic too; it can be hard to know where to put your feelings of frustration, injustice and despair when they have been wound up so tight to fuel getting a diagnosis in the first place. Take some time to think about your options, research and learn about the condition and various treatments. You don't always have to make a decision right away, and your doctors can help guide you based on *your* disease.

4
Why aren't we talking about it?

Endometriosis? Never heard of it!

It's said that 200 million women worldwide suffer from endometriosis, yet hardly anyone can tell you what it is, let alone pronounce it. But if it's as prevalent as arthritis and asthma why don't we all know about it?

There are lots of reasons why we don't talk about it and that can be hard to untangle. Is it because:

- it only affects women?
- it's embarrassing to talk about?
- we don't talk about periods full stop?
- we still believe that it's a 'woman's lot' to have pain or painful periods?
- we have been taught it is unattractive and unladylike to talk about our private parts anyway, but *especially* if something is wrong with them?

The problem is, if we don't talk about endometriosis more openly, people won't be aware of it, and without better awareness it's not only the disease that's invisible, but the millions of women who have it are too.

It's only very recently that awareness of the condition is increasing but it's still painfully slow; even those who have heard of it don't quite know what it actually is. It takes an average of seven to ten years to get a diagnosis and the treatments available are limited and often invasive. There aren't enough specialists, research is underfunded and because it's hard to get hold of accurate information a lot of myths continue to be perpetuated about this disease. But if no one knows about endometriosis and no one is talking about it, it won't get better. This silence and lack of awareness becomes a vicious cycle that leads to a delay in diagnosis and prolonged pain and suffering.

Endometriosis does not discriminate. It can affect women of any race, religion, sexuality and class; it's even believed Queen Victoria had it back in the day. As I navigate the health system, I am conscious that I have some privilege as a white, middle class woman who has been brought up believing I have a right to be heard, woman or not. My lack of embarrassment around this stuff, the fact that I'm not often intimidated by those in authority and that I am able to articulate how I feel also puts me at an advantage – but what about those who aren't like me? What if you're family never talk about such things? What if your culture or religion adds another layer of guilt or shame around periods and your body, which makes it impossible to speak up even when something feels wrong? What happens to the women who are quieter, meeker or more embarrassed? What if those women don't ever go to the doctor at all and *really* suffer in silence for much of their lives?

The period taboo

Emma Cox, CEO of Endometriosis UK, told me that two of their primary aims are to improve menstrual well-being education and remove the stigma around periods. They believe that increasing awareness of what is normal and what might not be, would help close the gap between initial symptoms and diagnosis.

In order to work out *why* we're not talking about endometriosis more, we have to start at the beginning – periods.

Most women have periods for a big chunk of our lives. They can be messy, inconvenient and, for some, painful, but we don't tend to talk about them much. We manage them quietly and without fuss, hiding tampons up sleeves, spending a fortune on period paraphernalia and generally keeping the complex bits of our bodies private. This goes on for about forty years and then when we stop menstruating and the menopause hits, guess what? We don't talk about that openly either (except for lame jokes about hot flushes). These major processes are going on in our bodies and we don't talk about them. It's odd isn't it? We see women's bodies all over the place all the time: we congratulate them when they deliver babies, we offer opinions on what we should do with them in terms of pubic hair or sexual fulfilment. We like the cleaned-up, cheeky talk about our bits but we don't like to talk about what *really* goes on, the *other* parts of our amazing parts.

My Wise Friend Alina

Alina is refreshingly open about periods, so I asked her why. She said, 'We're born alone and die alone but share most things with other humans, we might as well talk and compare when we can for comfort and advice. I'm not sure where I get my openness from. My parents aren't that open, my family is Indian and it's not something that they would talk about *ever*, but I'm an Aries so that might be it?'

She once told me that a perfect host should have tampons and pads in the toilet at a party as an act of solidarity. I love this idea, so I did it. There is now a box of 'sanitary delights' in my loo stuffed with everything you could ever want or need.

Q. What is the difference between menstruation and masturbation?

A. If you don't know the difference you shouldn't be doing either

When I was fourteen, us girls were taken to a science lab with an older, matronly biology teacher and the boys went to a regular classroom for a 'chat' with the young male PE teachers. In the lab, we huddled around the workbenches excited to hear about what our bits could *really* do, but instead we were given a mundane and muddled talk about periods, sex and contraception. Given we'd all started menstruating already it was pretty redundant teaching us about them then. Even the 'introduction to contraception' was pretty pointless, most had been 'introduced' some time ago (there wasn't much to do in Yorkshire in the early 1990s).

Luckily my mum had talked to me about periods before mine started, so it wasn't a shock, but even so, my adolescent body felt like a really complicated flat-packed item from IKEA with inadequate instructions and lots of little bits and bobs I had to work out on my own. I wasn't alone; all of us were somehow bumbling along with slightly wrong information from magazines, older sisters and cousins. We needed more information and support, and we deserved to have a better understanding of our bodies than this.

In the boys' classroom the male teachers said that the girls were talking about periods and then gave the advice: 'Don't look in a girl's handbag because she'll be embarrassed.' That's it. That's the sum total of what the boys learnt about menstruation, and women's genitals. The same ones they were created by, the same ones that many of them longed to be inside, the same ones they would spend the rest of their lives half knowing about. For the next hour they learnt how to put a condom on, using the extending handle of a window.

Splitting us up might appear to have been an act of kindness; protecting the girls from the jeers of teenage boys, allowing us to ask awkward questions and learn about what our bodies do in peace, but it also created a division. For the girls it reinforced the idea that periods *are* embarrassing and not something to talk about in front of boys, and the boys were essentially told that they didn't need to know about them at all. But doesn't *everyone* need to know this stuff? There's little point in knowing about osmosis or photosynthesis if we don't know how our own systems work. Teaching the girls, but not the boys, about menstruation and reproductive health made it 'women's problems' right there and then. It conditioned *everyone* that what happens in women's bodies is to be kept private.

Looking back, it also seems crazy to me to mix up menstruation, sex and fertility in one session; it unconsciously defines women by their reproductive abilities, which is insane when you consider I started my periods age eleven. Of course periods mark the beginning of fertility, and that is their biological function, but in terms of real life, this is not what we need to know most about. On average women have over four hundred periods in a lifetime, but may only have one to three children, if they have them at all. So shouldn't the focus be on menstrual well-being rather than the fertility bit? The lessons should include how we handle, manage and *live* with periods; what is normal and what isn't, what hormonal treatments are available and what they actually do, what items best soak up the blood, should we take painkillers for the cramps – if so, which ones are best? What do we do if we're still 'on' and we want to have sex? Can we take something to stop them for a bit, so we don't have the hassle when we're on holiday, or doing something important at work? Periods are more complicated than fertility alone and it should be taught that way, after all women spend much more time living with periods than without them.

Periods SSSSSSHHHHHH!

If we don't talk about periods how do we know what is 'normal' and what isn't? If your periods also come with a painful and complicated set of symptoms but you don't know that's not normal, it's likely you won't go and get help. The period taboo makes it harder for women to talk about endometriosis, or perhaps even know that such a thing exists. I didn't know it was a 'thing', I just assumed I was too sensitive, that other women managed period pain better and that's why no one talked about it. But mine weren't just 'bad periods'; it was endometriosis, a disease, and had I known more about periods, had people talked more, I might have recognised something was wrong and got help earlier.

THINGS I KNOW NOW

- Excessive period pain is not normal.

- Enduring pain is not just 'part of being a woman'.

- Periods shouldn't stop you from going to school, work or social activities.

- Endometriosis pain isn't the same as menstrual cramps; it's cramps on steroids.

- A good understanding of our bodies would help avoid all sorts of confusion and delays in seeking advice if something seems wrong (this goes for most things, not just endometriosis).

- Being ignorant about periods is a contributory factor in persistent myths and shame around menstruation, which can lead to delays in seeking help for something like endometriosis.

Periods aren't funny. Period.

So, we are conditioned from the beginning that periods are icky and private; they are *not* to be discussed in public but, if you really must, you should do it quietly. So, if we *do* talk about them it's in coy and pejorative terms; they're a burden, something to get through and something that happens *to* us not *in* us. I asked my women friends what they call their periods and here's what I got back:

On the blob/the blob	The curse
Man United are playing at home	Medea
Lady's time	Moon days
Carrie is here	I'm on/due on
On the rag	Aunt Flo is visiting
Shark week	Surfing the crimson wave
Time of the month	Monthlies
Got the painters in	Sister Mary is in the house
My time has come	Mother Nature's here

Some of these are pretty funny (and dark) but they're not particularly joyous or positive; in fact some are even a bit disturbing when you consider we're talking about a regular experience. I understand the desire to use euphemisms; that some women feel more comfortable using these terms over the accurate 'vulgar' terminology, but it's difficult to know whether these are *our* feelings about periods or if they have been created by a patriarchal society in which we all live. It might seem harmless and silly to focus in this but using pejorative language can unconsciously create or reinforce our sense of embarrassment about our bodies, and make it harder to discuss when things go wrong with them. As women we learn quickly that, however incredible our reproductive system is, the truths about it are to be hidden and if you talk about it you'll be oversharing and inappropriate. Perhaps *this* is why we are using these terms, adhering to this notion we should be quiet and socially acceptable on the rare occasions we do talk about such things.

A change is gonna come

The taboo around periods is getting better. Online campaigns such as #Periodpositive have increased awareness and broken down some of the stigma. In 2017, Bodyform made the first ever advert showing red liquid and not that ridiculous blue nonsense. (No wonder we've been confused for so long; we were led to believe menstrual blood should look like de-icer or a blueberry Slush Puppie.) Lobbying to end period poverty, where financial constraints leave young women unable to afford pads and tampons, has forced government to provide some free menstrual items in all secondary schools in England and opened up a much needed conversation around menstrual well-being generally.

In 2019, the Department for Education published new Draft Guidelines for Relationships, Health and Sex Education in schools. While revised and more liberal guidelines are to be welcomed (especially the inclusion of LGBTQ relationships), menstrual well-being and menstruation is not explicitly mentioned until secondary school level. Primary schools are expected to discuss puberty and changes in the adolescent body but if girls are starting to menstruate as young as eight, provision for managing periods as part of health and science education is clearly needed. The intention behind the reforms is to create a better understanding at a primary level, which is then built on at secondary.

However, as they remain guidelines, there is a still a chance that information may be diluted or adapted to placate the more conservative views of the school, teacher or community around them. It's not clear how periods will be talked about either – whether it will be included in health and science or only as part of sex education, linked to fertility and pregnancy. Ensuring useful, thorough and value free information is given to children relies on well-trained, confident teachers with time to prepare and deliver it. Anything that educates *everyone* and demystifies women's bodies is brilliant, especially if we are to increase awareness of women's health issues like endometriosis, but there is still a way to go.

Women are more open about our bodies than we have ever been, but there is still work to do and myths and embarrassment around periods remain. While we don't talk about them, are ashamed or even disgusted by them, and while they are regarded as something only *women* should be informed or bothered about, those who have conditions connected to them will continue to suffer in silence, perhaps even thinking it is their fault or that they are weak or abnormal.

It's not just periods though is it?

Endometriosis isn't just about menstruation. It can affect mental health, energy, immune function and these symptoms might also (confusingly) occur on a daily basis, so it's sort of about periods but it isn't at the same time.

It's my vagina and I'll call it what I want to!

So, we've already been conditioned not to talk about periods, but we don't talk about our private parts either, because it's inappropriate and you don't want to come across as brash, crass or slutty. So in addition to the quaint terms for periods, we come up with all sorts of names for our genitals too. Some are strong and bolshie for adults and some are more polite and metaphorical for children. But whatever we use they are designed to make it less embarrassing to discuss them.

Vulva	Vag	Front bottom
Muff	Cunt	Privates
Chuff	Vajayjay	Minnie
Lady bits	Pussy	Foo-foo
Fuff	Twat	Hoo-hee
My bits	Twinkle	Hoo-hoo (now you're
Vagina	Fan/ Fanny	just making sounds)

Everyone has a name for their parts, and this is all well and good. But what happens when something goes wrong with them and the doctor is too embarrassed to say the words too? Here are some of the terms I've heard from professional vagina merchants (or, as they're more commonly known, gynaecologists) over the years:

Tummy	Down below
Stomach	Nether regions
Downstairs	Front passage (as in where to
Abdomen	leave a parcel?)
Down there	

No wonder it takes so long to get anything diagnosed if everyone is confusing things by (literally) beating around the bush. Diagnostically, if they refer to your 'tummy' it could be anything! So, when they say this I think, 'Let's call a spade a spade, Doctor, you're not going to go in and operate on my 'tummy', you're going to cut and laser around my reproductive organs. You're going to release my stuck ovaries and get rid of this old blood sticking my uterus to my bowel and my Pouch of Douglas.' (I always think this sounds like a place to visit: 'We took a lovely boat trip around the Pouch of Douglas.')

Doctors aren't *actually* embarrassed by the real words, they may even be using these terms to put us at ease, but paradoxically when a doctor doesn't use the proper and specific words it can make the whole thing even more awkward. We start to talk in hushed tones and daren't say what's really happening in case it's perceived as vulgar or that we're bringing the tone down. It's important for *everyone* to be accurate and honest when we talk about symptoms as it helps doctors decipher what information is pertinent and this can be crucial in getting the right diagnosis and the *right* treatment.

It's embarrassing to talk about because it involves my bits

It's harder to talk about endometriosis than other long-term health conditions because it literally involves our private parts; personal things like periods, bowels and sex. It feels way more embarrassing to talk to colleagues, family members and potential lovers about this than it would be if you had diabetes or arthritis. My experience has also taught me that people are much more sympathetic about those other conditions because they know more about them, they're less embarrassed by them and can relate in some way. With endometriosis people seem to think it's just bad periods and they assume you should just 'Take a paracetamol and get on with it' like they do.

It's just 'women's problems'

There is an unspoken assumption from many, including some doctors (male and female), that a woman's lot is to have pain, and an expectation that we should suffer quietly and stop whining. After all, it's just 'women's problems'. We feel ashamed if we can't handle it, that we're complaining about something that all women go through. Even among women we can be made to feel like we're letting the side down by exposing something that makes us 'weaker'.

The catch-all term 'women's problems' is ridiculous as it covers anything that involves the female reproductive organs including periods, pregnancy complications, any postnatal effects, polycystic ovaries, fibroids, endometriosis, adenomyosis, infertility and ovarian and cervical cancers. These are all very different things. Some may have similar symptoms but they shouldn't be bunched together as a problem of gender. We don't talk about prostate or testicular cancer, low sperm count and erectile dysfunction as 'men's problems'. 'Women's problems' is a trivialising, nondescript term that reinforces a distasteful view that women are fussing. It allows us to ignore, undermine or 'normalise' women's pain, the complexity of our bodies and the far-reaching impact these conditions can have on the rest of our lives. Such terminology serves only to silence and disregard women's suffering and it doesn't help individuals in the pursuit of a diagnosis for something like endometriosis. The complicity in this misogynist view of women is perpetuated by an undereducated medical system, and as patients we are conditioned to collude in it.

We apologise for visiting a doctor yet again to ask what might be wrong, we let them leave us lolling on chairs in A&E because it's just 'period pain' and we've sort of come to believe that ourselves. We get used to the pain and the dismissal and then we're too tired or jaded to fight back. Even now, after over twenty years of living with endometriosis, I delay asking for help for fear that someone will suggest I'm fussing or overreacting. This put-up and shut-up attitude must be contributing to the delays in diagnosis and better treatments for endometriosis long term.

Even if 'women's problems' *were* only affecting women, our experiences shouldn't be dismissed. We're half of the population. But these are not just issues for women; they have an impact on those around us too. 'Women's problems' are everyone's problem. While endometriosis is a female disease (as it only physically affects women), as a society we are *all* affected by it: employers, the economy, the health system, the emotional and financial effects on friends, lovers and family. This disease doesn't just affect the individual, so it needs to be better understood and discussed by society and, even more critically, within the medical profession so as to reduce the dismissive, lazy and inaccurate assumptions made by us all regarding 'women's problems'.

Awareness is the key

Every expert I've spoken to agreed that better awareness is the key to it all. If doctors are given more training about endometriosis, they will be better equipped to help women reach diagnosis and treatment quicker. If women are more aware of it they will seek help and treatment earlier from the right sources. If *all* of us in society were better informed about women's bodies and health issues, it would not only help women with endometriosis, but also those around them too: at her work, her school, in her family. Everyone would be more tolerant and supportive of the effects of this condition. The lack of urgency to improve awareness is perhaps because it isn't life-threatening, but it can be *life-changing* or *life-reducing* if it isn't managed properly. If more people knew about this disease and just how *many* women are affected, surely there would be more demand to fund vital research that would undoubtedly increase the chances of better treatments to modify the disease, less invasive ways to diagnose, a better understanding of the disease and maybe, just maybe, one day even a cure.

Things We Can Do Now to Make Awareness Better

- **Better menstrual health education for ALL**: would reduce the taboo and allow everyone to talk more openly.
- **Educate medical practitioners at *all levels***: warning signs, symptoms, treatments, building awareness of referral pathways to the right support.
- **Review our approach to 'women's problems'**: change opinions of women's pain and health in the medical community and wider society: schools, work environments, in our personal lives.
- **Train more endometriosis specialists, sonographers, surgeons, pelvic pain and hormonal experts**: if such doctors were in *all* hospitals it would change perceptions and increase awareness. Endometriosis would become a standard thing, treated like other conditions, not an obscure specialism.

- **Stop perpetuating myths**: if you don't know, don't speculate (and get educated).
- **Increase funding for research**: enable cohesive, wider studies that include input from thousands of women and doctors.
- **Encourage autonomy among patients while also providing support**: inform, educate, explain options and prognosis. Give women the tools to manage living with it. Then we can tackle it together.

5
Gender bias and endometriosis

What if men had endometriosis?

I often wonder if men had endometriosis might we know more about it? I don't think the sole reason it's being overlooked is because it only affects women, but it's worth asking if men were suffering too would a greater amount of money, time and research be allocated to it? I asked Professor Krina Zondervan, Co-director of the Endometriosis CaRe Centre at Oxford University, if she thought the fact this is a female disease is a contributory factor to its neglect in terms of research and funding:

> I think it's one factor. Because it affects only women there may also be a reticence and shyness, to talk about it and the symptoms that come with it. If people don't talk about how it affects some people, there's not enough incentive for funding bodies who respond to economic cost pictures and I think it is only more recently that this has been highlighted. This is a cost to society, not just a health care cost, which includes the cost of women not

being able to work or fulfill other daily activities. The research statistics are pretty shocking, especially when you consider type two diabetes is nearly as prevalent and has a similar picture in terms of health care cost. It has been reported that the National Institutes of Health (the main governmental research funding body in the US) spends approximately 36 dollars a year per patient in grant money on diabetes, but for endometriosis less than a dollar.

The really cynical part of me says that it is precisely *because* it only affects women that it is not taken as seriously as diabetes or asthma, which have similar numbers of sufferers but receive more funding and awareness because these conditions also affect men. If men were unable to work or were in pain on a monthly basis, if they were debilitated and only being offered invasive and (for some) intolerable treatments then I think the urgency to find better solutions would be greater. One can't help but wonder if the lack of motivation to really investigate, talk about and change the situation for women with this condition is connected to how we value women and their contribution to society. But it's also important to remember that, and this is the tragic irony, women are contributing to the silence around this condition too. It's more pernicious than just disinterest because it only affects women; the patriarchal society in which we all live means that women are taught and conditioned to perceive 'women's problems' as being secret and so we don't talk about them either.

Endometriosis, and its lack of research, satisfactory treatments and outcomes, is a feminist issue. But it is possible to break down taboos around female health conditions. The awareness and open discussion of something like breast cancer for example has increased hugely in the last twenty years due to women speaking up, targeted campaigns and a lot of work. We need to do the same for other female health issues that may feel awkward to talk about.

Women's pain

There is a gender bias, both in society and in the medical profession, when it comes to how women are treated in terms of pain. Studies have shown that men are less likely to be told that their pain is psychological and are more likely to be prescribed and given pain relief quicker than women, because there remains an assumption that if a man is speaking up about his pain he must be in agony, but a woman must be overreacting. I don't know about you, but every woman I know would rather be anywhere else on a Saturday night than A&E. My bet is she's done everything she can to stop this being the outcome. The women I know who suffer with pain or any physical complaint usually don't talk about it much and when they do, they're dismissive of their experiences and laugh it off. But stereotypes remain strong: men are stoic and silent and women show their feelings or are more 'in tune' with their bodies so they are more likely to seek medical advice more often and quicker.

Women are conditioned to question themselves because of these stereotypes and the traditional medical system reinforces this, putting women at a disadvantage. The NICE guidelines on endometriosis said medical practitioners needed 'to listen to women more'. This was also the belief of every endometriosis specialist I have spoken to. They all agreed that one of the best ways to understand the disease, reach diagnosis and treat effectively is to look at the woman in front of them not a textbook or a bunch of tests. *Talking* about the individual's symptoms and life is vital, as a few questions can tell you much more about their experience each month than a blood test or surgery. Yet for many women with endometriosis this level of consultation is rarely realised, and we are often dismissed in our quest for diagnosis and help.

The intricacy of women's complex reproductive systems, and therefore the many things that can go wrong with various bits of them, suggests that they, of all people, shouldn't be dismissed. That's why there's a whole medical discipline, gynaecology, just for these organs. But what happens when you meet gynaecologists and *they* dismiss you too?

She's crazy

Historically, women's pain has often been dismissed as psychological, hysterical or hormonal; particularly when unable to explain a cause. I often wonder if this idea has disappeared or whether it lingers unconsciously in the medical (and society's) approach to female pain. Hysteria comes from the Greek word for womb and I hate it. It is a leftover word from a male history; another umbrella term for an indefinable neurotic illness from a time where medicine approached everything through a male lens. Traditionally science viewed the male body as 'normal' or the status quo to which a woman's body was compared and seen in relation to, and as such any differences were perceived as 'abnormal'. Some believed women's bodies were 'missing' the male parts or that we had inverted male organs, or that women's wombs travelled around their bodies and dictated their behaviour. Some even thought wombs made women unbalanced and 'hysteria' explained heightened emotional states or abnormal sexual desire (like wanting or 'over-enjoying' sex).

Its meaning has changed a bit since then. Mostly we use it to describe something very funny, but its original usage is still alive and well, often used to suggest that someone's behaviour is out of control and crazy – and usually that someone is female. Indeed as late as the 1980s, women with endometriosis talk of being diagnosed with psychosis and their experiences dismissed, some were given unnecessary hysterectomies because no one knew what else to do or because by the time someone took them seriously the disease was so advanced it was unavoidable. I don't get angry much, but if someone calls me hysterical I, ironically, want to punch them in the face and tip a table. The notion is that I have no capacity for reason or logic; that my womb or hormones are making me overreact. For me the implication that women are unable to control their behaviour because of their bodies, and my fear of being labelled 'hysterical', has been a large part of why I kept quiet about having this condition. Although endometriosis and luck have not aligned much in my life, I feel very lucky to have been born in a time where I have more rights as a woman than those before me and perceptions of women's pain have adapted somewhat, where doctors haven't just slammed me into a mental institution, sedated me or whipped out my uterus and told me it's all in my head. However, despite having encountered many brilliant doctors, I have also experienced the doubt, dismissal and disbelief of some. I have been given the wrong information or been fobbed off, scorned for being intelligent, as though this in itself might be making the situation worse – 'Don't worry yourself so much.' I have often been told that it is my emotional state that's the problem, not the fact I have a physical disease and I have often felt crazy or mad when I'm trying to work out how I'm going to actually *live* with endometriosis.

THINGS I KNOW NOW

- The doctors who have operated on me or helped me make major treatment decisions don't doubt or dismiss, they advise with sound medical knowledge based on what is best for me. If there is any sign of misogyny I see it as a red light, an indicator that I need to leave and never see that doctor again.

- It can be difficult to walk away if you believe this is the *one* person who might be able to help you, but if you have doubts find another doctor. You're too important.

Has it changed?

I'm in no doubt that the majority of medical professionals are kind, intelligent and open-minded, but this doesn't exclude the possibility that they approach their work with their own set of beliefs and experiences. While medicine has become more advanced in techniques and thinking, it doesn't mean that the beliefs around 'women's problems' and women's pain have been entirely eradicated. If hysteria was the framework for 'women's problems', we need to be diligent that such views aren't creeping back in. As with any societal and political shift, just because something is no longer deemed acceptable doesn't mean attitudes have actually *changed*. Even if such beliefs are unconscious it's possible that an insidious misogyny remains and this gender bias may impact how you are treated.

Girl-on-girl crime

The large majority of gynaecologists I have met are men who specialise in specifically female conditions that they can never actually have themselves. This isn't a problem in itself; doctors don't have to experience something themselves to be able to treat it. But it might make it harder to empathise with the effects of the treatments they're offering or to have a more sympathetic approach to their patients with endometriosis. However, what is surprising, and perhaps one of the saddest things I've experienced, is that almost all of the female gynaecologists I have met have been the least compassionate of all. This is weird, right? Their experience of menstruation or 'women's problems' should make them more sympathetic, not less. So when *they* doubt that the pain is real or assume we're exaggerating, when they imply that we *all* have to deal with this stuff so stop complaining, it can be even more upsetting. The feeling when this happens is not just disappointment, it's a gut drop. You thought there was a sister-hood, that they, more than anyone, would understand or, at the very least, believe you, and then you feel hopeless because if *they* don't get this then who will?

I sometimes wonder if the misogyny that underpins how we approach 'women's problems' contributes to why women are less tolerant of each other in these situations. It's also worth considering that although there are more women in medical roles than ever, they are part of a traditionally male world of medicine, and the systemic 'male' perspective is hard to change. Medicine is not exclusive in this regard; there are still many areas where women may feel they cannot afford to be sympathetic to each other if they are to get ahead in a 'male' environment.

As a caveat, I have also met some great female doctors and the women in my life are brilliant, caring, patient and understanding. I hope you've found more of them in your journey than the doctors I'm talking about above.

6
Talking about it with others

I used to think there were only two ways to manage living with endometriosis: totally secret (apart from a few trusted people) or blabbing about it to anyone and using it as an excuse or identity. I was wrong. Although I was reluctant to talk about it for a long time, when the symptoms became more difficult to manage, I had to become more open and mostly I have found people to be much more understanding than I thought they would be. I've learnt that there are many ways to live with endometriosis and whether you talk about it or not is an important part of it.

THINGS I KNOW NOW

Being more open might help but you may have to decide *how*, *where* and *to whom*.

- It may be that certain people can't deal with the complexity and inconsistency of the disease; they don't understand why you can't make it to something when you seemed fine yesterday or why it isn't 'fixed' yet.

- It may be that your employers would be less than under-standing and you would miss out on a promotion or you'd even lose that job.

- It may be that you don't want it to affect your sexual relationship by talking about it in depth; you want those parts of you to be alluring and exciting, not painful and vulnerable.

Whatever you choose will be right for you and if what you choose stops working, you can adapt your approach.

So how do we talk about it?

There doesn't appear to be a genetic component for me, no one in my family seems to have suffered from it. I look at my wonderful nieces, their joyful faces, little bodies and carefree movements and can't bear the thought that they would have to experience *any* kind of pain, let alone this disease. Sometimes I hope that the reason why I have such a horrible version is so I can swallow it up, that it will live and die with me. But the fact I didn't know anyone with endometriosis for a long time meant it was hard to communicate what it was really like to live with it to those around me. A general ignorance about the condition, perpetuation of myths and that it's part of 'women's problems' can also make people embarrassed or more likely to dismiss it. It may also be that there are cultural reasons for some women to keep quiet about it, or those around you consider it to be inappropriate to discuss anything to do with menstruation or female 'private parts'. But I believe there is a difference between being private and personal and something being too taboo to discuss. It's about finding a balance that you feel comfortable with, so people understand but you don't feel exposed or 'not normal'.

Finding the words

It can be difficult to articulate what endometriosis *feels* like, especially when you are actually in the middle of *feeling* it and it's also hard to explain a non-visible illness as we have to rely on words to express it. One of the ways the doctors have helped me is to use a pain-management technique where you visualise the disease and try to put into words what it feels and looks like. It gives you back some control and enables you to explain an invisible illness to those who are struggling to understand. It's a useful and empowering exercise – maybe try it too?

What Does It Feel Like?

At its worst you feel heavy and miserable, like you're about to get the flu. It's like a combination of a dodgy tummy, backache and vomiting.

It's an aching in your legs, your lower abdomen and even weirdly in the back of your throat; a sort of metallic nausea.

Your abdomen swells and you feel like you're holding litres of water.

Sometimes it feels like being kicked in the vagina. Sometimes it feels like it might all fall out.

Sometimes all you can do is sleep or curl up and wait for it to pass; sometimes you can fight through and make it to that party, hoping the oxytocin will abate the pain and wake you up a little.

Sometimes it's so painful you want to pass out – and sometimes you do.

Oh, and you're always so very tired.

Invisible

Because you can't *see* it, it's harder for others to believe and make sense of what you're going through. For a long time, I liked the fact that it was an invisible illness, that I mostly didn't *look* ill. On the days I did, make-up hid the dark lines under my eyes and the pale, green skin. I got to decide what I could and couldn't manage. But the downside of it being invisible is that it makes it harder for people to get what all the fuss is about. If it's a broken leg, people can see it and you recover from it. But you can't see endometriosis, and you don't really 'recover'; you learn to manage and live with it. When it comes to acute illnesses like colds, sore throats and flu, people understand these because they can see them, they've experienced them, they're easy to explain and label, there is a pain level attributed to them and, most importantly, there is a treatment that works and an end point. People lose their shit when there isn't an end point, they don't know how to react to long-term conditions that don't have a cure.

I don't like that it's invisible when . . .

. . . people don't recognise it takes time to recover from operations; it might be keyhole but it *is* major surgery.

. . . I have to repeatedly explain myself to people who don't see what the problem is, why it isn't it fixed yet? (As though it's a verruca I've been too lazy to sort out.)

. . . I have to decide whether the symptoms are bearable today, because if I turn up people assume I must be OK and sometimes I'm not and my body says 'Na-ah'.

I wish people could see endometriosis sometimes. From the outside it looks smooth, round – normal (apart from a bunch of tiny surgical scars) but underneath . . .

What does it look like?

I imagine heavy stones hanging precariously in an empty room with thickly painted dark cerise walls and a high ceiling. I imagine the embers and charcoal like the fire at my grandmother's, dusty and hot. I imagine a battle scene in *Lord of the Rings* – a dark and bumpy terrain with little burning fires all over the place.

When the pain is really bad I imagine a giant cartoon lever that is stuck on 'on'. I think of tiny people inside who work as technicians managing the messages between the body and brain. I envisage loads of them dangling off the lever, pulling down on it and trying to turn it off. These little people don't look like me, they don't have big bottoms and long brown hair, they're sort of fuzzy and nondescript. They're doing their best but it isn't good enough, it's mayhem in there; alarms going off, vats of stuff tipped over and oozing every- where like the green slime at the end of *Who Framed Roger Rabbit*. But it's not slime, it's blood, and it's got nowhere to go and although tools and big hands (think *Honey I Shrunk the Kids*) might come in and try and clean it up once in a while, the floors won't ever be quite the same. There'll be dried stuff in the corners and a bit behind something that will get missed; there are stains on the floor of my abdomen that can't be removed.

Then it's calm again, back to little embers and smoke from a not-quite-forgotten crisis.

Bored!

Although living with endometriosis sometimes includes moments of drama, going to A&E or having surgery, the day-to-day manage- ment can begin to bore everyone, including you after some time. The long-term nature of this condition can make it more difficult for others to sustain interest or even sympathy sometimes. They may be impatient that it hasn't been resolved or feel they have nothing left to say or do to help. By my eighth surgery it had become so 'normal' for me that my friends and family asked what time I was going in as though it were a haircut. We had *all* forgotten that operations aren't a common thing in most people's lives.

How to handle unhelpful input

Over the years I have learnt to manage my frustration (and fists) when others, usually with no direct experience, offer advice.

Some Unhelpful Things People Say (All the Time)

- Do you have painful sex then?
- Does that mean you can't have children?
- You can always adopt though can't you?
- I know how you feel – I have terrible periods!
- Why don't you have a baby? That's a cure.
- Do you think the painkillers are actually *doing* anything?
- You came to that party last night, what's wrong with you today?
- What is the plan here? You can't go on like this!
- Often it's all in your head you know.
- It's just bad periods, nothing that can be done!
- Are you just going to have done with it and get it all taken out?
- Do you think you're just hypersensitive?
- Can't you just mentally override it?
- Do you still have that?

What might be surprising is that even doctors have said some of these things to me over the years! It's tiresome to smile and listen to the quasi-cures and myths, but I now adopt this policy: *no endometriosis, no opinion.* If the person talking to you has no real understanding of this disease and the potential effects on your physical and emotional well-being, but insists on suggesting something you know won't work, you can enlighten and educate them, suggest they read up about it themselves, or just say 'Thanks, I'll try that' and leave.

THINGS I KNOW NOW

If people aren't kind and supportive when you explain why you can't come to something, or they diminish or dismiss your experience, walk away. It is *their* problem, not yours. It may be hard to lose these people from your life but it's surprising who steps up when it gets hard; they're often the people you least expect and they're usually the most wonderful.

A friend of mine had that . . .

Sometimes people casually mention that their friend, or cousin's friend's sister, got rid of their endometriosis by running or by having a baby. Once someone told me that their friend had cured hers with mint tea. Was it a special kind? Peppermint or spearmint? Did she get some magic beans while she was at it? Mostly people are trying to be helpful, and it often comes from a kind place, but it can feel like they are saying: why haven't you tried this? What have you been *actively* doing to solve it? This person is managing much better than you, why haven't you *tried* to get better?

It can be very dispiriting when people don't seem to grasp that this is something which doesn't have 'a fix' and you have to spend time (and precious energy) persuading them that you're doing everything you can to feel as well as possible, to not let the symptoms control your life, while simultaneously trying to manage the symptoms which are, in fact, sometimes controlling your life.

THINGS I KNOW NOW

- When explaining endometriosis to someone, try to liken the symptoms to something they might have experienced; e.g. the worst period pain you can think of, plus food poisoning and backache.

- One friend told me about the pelvic pain she had when she was pregnant. I gently mentioned it sounded very similar; she's been more sympathetic since!

I've had that . . .

A funny feeling when you *do* talk about endometriosis is that you want to feel as if you have the worst version of it; maybe people will take it more seriously if it's *really* bad. Perhaps the competitive nature of this particular illness is because we have often been suffering privately for so long that, when we do get a chance to talk about it, we need to be heard. We want our endurance to be recognised and praised. This competitive behaviour can often be found in online forums, or when an acquaintance tells you of someone they know who has it much worse than you. It can be difficult to find the line between people trying to be supportive and sharing their experience, and this competition. The woe-is-me, mine-is-worse attitude is also particularly hard to be around when you're just about holding it together yourself. But there is no room for this competition. It's not useful for anyone, everything should be in context and no one who has endometriosis is having a nice time.

THINGS I KNOW NOW

Laughter is the best medicine. (Morphine is a strong contender.)

Laughing is one of the best coping strategies you can have with a frustrating and ever-changing condition like endometriosis. It can be reassuring. It makes the insane saner. It's a release. I haven't always been a comedian, but humour has always helped me with hard situations. I don't feel the need to do it all the time but making light of it helps to diffuse the tension and allows me to process to the important information without crying in a heap right there in the doctor's office, (I can do that after!) I've learned that it's vital to see the world outside of the illness, to remember life is about more than this and finding the laughs wherever possible helps you to stay optimistic and gives you some control over it all.

Talking to lovers

You can lose your sense of sexuality when your gubbins are the source of pain and trauma and if you're not in a loving relationship this can be tricky to explain to new lovers. Sometimes sexual desire is not affected at all but it's just difficult to meet someone or go on dates when you spend a lot of time feeling poorly. If you're single there may also be fears of 'Who wants to be lumbered with this?' creeping in, especially if you're having a bad patch, when even the *idea* of dating can be overwhelming.

It can also be hard to know how and when to tell a potential partner about it. Common fears are that simply saying you have endometriosis may mean you are no longer perceived as desirable or sexy, or they'll freak out. But something I know now is that if this is the case, they aren't worthy of you anyway. Another concern is that if it affects fertility you have a moral obligation to share this; but do you *know* this is the case for you?

For many years I didn't tell partners until I had to. I had anxieties about how they might respond but mostly there were plenty of other things to talk about. During the times when it was a bigger part of my life but I didn't want to say anything, I used a half-truth. One time I'd just started dating a guy when I had to have another surgery. I wasn't ready to talk to him about it, so I told him I had an ovarian cyst, which was the truth but not the whole truth. Crucially I got to choose when I shared it and how. This is a significant part of how I cope with living with endometriosis; because there is still so much confusion and misunderstanding around the condition, it's very important to me to be able to control how I explain *my* version of it, on my terms.

I can't tell you *when* to tell someone but I can tell you that I don't think there is an obligation to talk about it any earlier than you want to. Having endometriosis isn't the defining thing about you; it's something you have and that you're living with. Ask yourself: do they need to know right now? Or maybe consider it another way: would you tell them you had another long-term health issue like a heart condition, asthma or diabetes on the first date?

Talking to work

For a long time I operated on a need-to-know basis. Close colleagues knew that this was something I had to deal with so they were understanding if I needed time off for surgeries and flare-ups, but I was managing it well enough to commit to the work I had agreed to do. I knew what I could handle and I never let anyone down so I felt this was the right approach. My determination to be successful helped me to endure the pain and hide quite how poorly I felt a lot of the time. It was my Achilles womb, but a private part of my life. I was also working with men a lot of the time and I didn't want to be treated differently; asking for help, for concessions or showing any weakness was not something I wanted to do in my working life, especially if the reason I might need that support was directly connected to being a woman.

Another major fear was that in a competitive industry, I wouldn't get acting jobs if they thought I was unreliable, so even mentioning it might mean the decision was taken out of my hands. When talking to other women in showbiz with endometriosis, this discretion so as to avoid people making assumptions about our capabilities doesn't stop however high up you get. One high-profile woman who agreed to be interviewed for this book later backed out because she worried that 'coming out' might hinder her work chances and eligibility for insurance at work. Misunderstanding and lack of sympathy around women's health issues really needs to be addressed, and quickly, if we feel even *talking* about such things will lead to penalisation in a work environment.

It's not uncommon to want keep your health issues private at work, and this is especially the case for many women with endometriosis because it's such a personal condition. It can feel inappropriate to mention it because of the parts involved and we don't want to be labelled with 'women's problems'. Another worry is what response we will get: will our employer be sympathetic and understanding? Or will this be used to undermine our work because we have this 'hormonal thing' they don't understand? Although it's discriminatory to penalise *anyone* for having a health condition, to get rid of you or pass you over for promotion, it does happen sometimes. It happened to me in one of my more conventional jobs when I had to tell them because I needed a considerable amount of time off to recover.

If you're managing fine you may you not need to let anyone know. But some women have no choice if they are experiencing flare-ups, new symptoms from a change in treatment or need time off for surgery. If you don't let your employer know, it can make it harder for them to be understanding and supportive when you need them to be. Confiding in your employer may in fact make your life easier. Perhaps they can offer flexible hours, working from home, occupational-health adjustments in the workplace and be more generally sympathetic. Whatever you decide in terms of managing your working life and endometriosis will be right for you. My instinct has always been that you don't *have* to tell anyone, especially if it isn't affecting your day-to-day life. This applies to work, lovers, friends, anyone, but you may require more support at particular times and sometimes telling people helps.

THINGS I KNOW NOW

To reduce anxiety around sick leave and what support you're entitled to it's hugely beneficial to seek legal advice or speak to your HR department, so you can be fully aware of your rights as an employee with a long-term health condition.

How do I research and find support?

There are lots of ways to find information about endometriosis, but it can be hard to know where to start and when you do it might feel overwhelming. There is a spectrum of suffering with this condition: some have milder symptoms that can be managed, some have difficulty finding the right treatment for them and others might be debilitated by the symptoms or the effects of the treatments. Because endometriosis affects everyone differently, it might be tricky to find the right information for *you* without being alarmed by others' experiences.

Books
There are a lot of books now. Some are a bit dry or written in medical jargon, but there are also some great, user-friendly books that discuss treatment options, their effects and efficacy (some are listed at the back of *this* book).

Online
In many ways my online access being so limited when I was first diagnosed was a blessing, as it allowed me to remain naive in the

beginning and avoid seeing some of the more distressing stories about the condition. But over the years I've used the Internet a lot to research treatments, and specialists, and find support and advice from other women.

The websites of organisations like Endometriosis UK or the Endometriosis Foundation of America are really good places to start (see page 342). Because of their charitable status they can only provide medically accurate information, so you won't find much about complementary medicine or radical ways to manage it, but their content is reliable and current. These sites are well organised, easy to navigate and positive in tone. They also provide links to local support groups, online groups and helpful advice for loved ones.

THINGS I KNOW NOW

Warning, these images might be distressing.

The Internet can be hugely beneficial for connecting women with endometriosis and researching treatments, but there are also lots of myths, quasi-cures and links to cowboy practitioners to be found too. If you've just been diagnosed or are struggling to manage your own condition, being faced with frightening images and accounts from strangers can sometimes be very upsetting. So here are some tips to help you navigate searching online:

- We're not all the same. Everyone experiences and approaches endometriosis differently; many women don't share their stories online – maybe because they are managing fine or they'd rather not share it this way. Try to remember that no one's experience is a definitive or inevitable version of this disease.

• Recognise that many sites are not medically regulated, so they may be inaccurate or perpetuating misunderstandings of the disease.

• When it comes to medical intervention remember that what works for one person might not for another (and vice versa).

• Don't read and click aimlessly, keep checking in with how you *feel*; it shouldn't make you more anxious.

• Ask a trusted friend or family member to vet a website if you're worried about what you might find.

Support groups

Many women gain strength and reassurance by talking to others with endometriosis. Websites like Health Unlocked provide a platform to discuss treatments and concerns and there is a real sense of community. But be aware these are patient testimonies and not always medically accurate. There are also blogs, Instagram, Twitter and Facebook accounts dedicated to endometriosis, where fellow 'endo-sisters' share inspirational articles, advice and stories. In real life there are support groups who meet up to talk or have guest speakers who share their expertise. Many of the local groups are run through the main charities in your country and there is usually a link to them on their websites (some of these are listed at the back of the book).

I can't handle someone else's story as well.

It can take time to come to terms with your diagnosis and fully absorb what it might mean for you. If you're over-whelmed with questions and worries about your own situation, it might feel impossible to empathise or engage with other people's experiences at this stage. That's OK. It doesn't make you a selfish person, so no guilt for this. But meeting other women with endometriosis can also be hugely beneficial, especially if you feel no one understands what it's like to live with it, if you're unsure about what happens next, or if you don't have people around to talk to. Groups can be very helpful for some and even if they might not be right for you at certain times, know that they are there if you need extra help at different stages of your life. You might even learn something new, meet some lifelong friends or find inspiration and comfort.

Building your support network

If you don't have close family or friends around, enquire about the Patient Advice and Liaison Service (PALS) at your hospital. This is a support and advocate service that helps patients navigate the health system and someone from the team may even be able to attend appointments with you.

Enquire about specialist endometriosis nurses too, their support has been invaluable to me over the years. They have extraordinary knowledge, expertise and kindness and can help with the right referral pathways, explain in more detail if you're confused about what the doctor said and guide you towards local or online support groups. If you have a BSGE accredited endometriosis centre at your hospital, ask if you can have an appointment with one of the specialist nurses.

7
A guide for the lads, dads, lovers, mothers and friends

It might be hard to explain how endometriosis is affecting you to people in your life, but they might also be struggling to know how they can help. It's also not uncommon to feel particularly awkward talking about this stuff, particularly with male relatives or friends. So if you're too tired, confused, or new to all this, or perhaps you've been living with it for a while and are sick of trying to explain it, fold down the corner of this page and hand the book to the person you love. I used to find it hard to talk about too, but not any more. Let me have a go.

Someone I love has endometriosis. What can I do?

- **Learn about it**: even an hour of (the right) research can be invaluable and useful for a lifetime. It will also stop you suggesting things that aren't helpful or aren't going to work.
- **Be curious, try to imagine what it's like**: this isn't 'just period

pain', this condition can cause extreme pain and a myriad of other symptoms.

- **Understand that a diagnosis can be a bit overwhelming**: there can be a lot of information to absorb, and it can be trial and error to find the right treatment.
- **Talk and listen to her**: she might not want (or be able) to articulate what she feels but let her know she can talk about it whenever she wants. Ask what is worrying her most. There are suddenly lots of things to think about: fertility concerns, hormonal changes that come with treatments and accepting she has something that needs to be managed and doesn't have a cure. This can be scary.
- **Be there for her**: a strong support network is vital. It's as important as the treatments the doctors are offering. They see her for ten minutes every six months, you see her all the time.
- **Believe her**: she needs you to know the pain is real. If you suggest she ought to just 'get on with it' or 'muster through' you will discourage her from sharing the physical and emotional pain that can come with this condition and it will make her feel more isolated and weird.
- **Be her advocate**: if she asks you to come to an appointment, ask how you can be helpful, whether that's being vocally supportive, taking notes or just sitting out in the waiting room.
- **Be in her corner**: it's possible the journey to diagnosis or a manageable treatment plan will be more difficult than we'd all hope. There may be times where she will need you to be stronger and fight for her if she is being dismissed or is simply too poorly to do it alone.
- **Be supportive**: there may be times when the symptoms are manageable and she decides to do something 'reckless'. If

these choices then cause a 'spike' in symptoms, don't say 'I told you so'.

- **Be patient**: each person handles this their own way; they may make mistakes or botch their way through. Try not to be too judgemental.
- **Be kind**: Sometimes you won't know what to say or do, but just saying 'It's unfair and horrible and I'm sorry you have to go through this' is enough. Recognition and kindness help enormously when you're struggling.

Practical stuff

- Ask what you can do to help.
- Tell her she's amazing to be handling it all and give her a cuddle.
- Make food and plenty of drinks.
- Provide comfort – baths, hot-water bottles, electric blankets.
- Give her some company – watch something together, sit with her, lie with her, play some music.
- There may be points in the month when extra support and being particularly conscientious would be useful.
- Help manage her world; not being able to do menial tasks can be very frustrating. You can help by doing some of these things.

What can I do longer term?

- **Don't avoid her**: it's lonely enough being in pain and feeling poorly, losing your social life, family and things to look forward to makes it so much bleaker.
- **Don't make decisions on her behalf**: keep inviting her to things. She will decide what she's capable of doing.
- **Don't treat her differently**: *she* hasn't changed.

- **Provide distraction**: talking, watching a film or box set together, a short walk or a meal out, read books out loud, take a little trip out of the house.
- **Encourage her**: when she tries to make lifestyle changes like diet or gentle exercise they can be hard to persist with.
- **Laughing is really important**: it might not fix it but it can really help when you feel hopeless.
- **Listen if she wants to talk**: just be there with her if she doesn't.
- **Send a text, go round for coffee, ring or FaceTime/Skype**: remind her she's missed when she can't come to something. Suggest what you might be able to do together instead.
- **Research, read and be active**: do these things when she can't, encourage her to find ways to manage it for herself but don't push this on her; when she's ready she will approach lifestyle changes such as diet, pacing (see page 204) and exercise.

This one goes out to the lovers

Your partner may be the one experiencing the symptoms, but it is important for you to be honest about how you feel too (but try not to be unnecessarily cruel). If you are worried about intimacy, or whether you can handle it all, find a way of discussing it and think about what *you* can do or suggest what might improve the situation. Remember that she is learning how to handle this too and it may take time to get control over the symptoms. Recognising the effects this might be having on your relationship is important, but how you communicate with each other about this is vital.

8
Surgical treatment

Once you know more about endometriosis and have become familiar with your own disease, the next stage is managing it in the best way possible for you. It may be that you can also make some life-style choices that will help to alleviate the symptoms and reduce medical intervention, but we'll come to that later.

What are my medical options?

There are various treatments available to manage the disease and symptoms and you may need to try a few until you get the right one for you. Remember we all experience different symptoms and respond to the treatments differently too. The medical options available currently are surgery or hormonal treatments and both present their own risks and side effects.

- **Surgery**: laparoscopy with laser/excision. Surgery is the only way to *remove* disease.
- **Hormonal treatments**: these may include the contraceptive pill, Mirena coil (IUD) or Depo-Provera injection, which are used to suppress disease growth and help you to manage the symptoms and your menstrual cycle.
- **Stronger hormone treatments**: GnRH analogue injections or tablets (Lupron and Zoladex are brand names you might have heard?) They create a pseudo-menopause. It isn't permanent and only lasts while you're on the treatment. You may also take add-back HRT (hormone replacement therapy) to protect bone density and reduce some of the side effects.
- **More radical surgery**: sometimes women might have a hysterectomy or partial hysterectomy but it is worth remembering that this is not necessarily a cure and should not be done lightly. It is non-reversible and comes with other risks and symptoms. You *must* discuss this with an endometriosis specialist and whenever possible seek more than one opinion.
- **How to find out more**: to learn about what the above medical treatments involve, other medical treatments, side effects and how they're administered through authorised websites like Endometriosis UK and The Endometriosis Foundation of America or in some of the books listed at the end of this book (see page 343)

Your doctor may suggest hormonal rather than surgical intervention initially, or that post-surgery, you have some form of hormone treatment to manage the disease and symptoms. They may also be able to offer you further support: the right pain medication; help with digestion, nausea, sleep and bowel issues. They can also help with referrals to physiotherapists, psychotherapists or pain specialists should you need this additional support.

Why surgery?

It is often difficult to establish the presence of endometriosis definitively without surgery. Depending on the type of disease you have it might be possible to see it on a scan, but this requires a specialist sonographer with expert understanding and training in endometriosis.

Surgery can be a lifeline for many women; it can reduce pain and severe symptoms. However, it's important to recognise that it has some risks and it doesn't always work. The disease can still grow back and even after extensive surgery the adhesions and scar tissue post-op can sometimes cause pain too. I spoke to consultant gynaecologist and endometriosis and fertility expert Michael Dooley:

> A good surgeon knows when to operate. A brilliant one knows when *not* to operate. It's very easy to do a surgery and people think you're wonderful, but actually it might not be right for the patient. A skilful surgeon knows when not to do it. We need to be careful not to medicalise it and treat the individual rather than the disease.

THINGS I KNOW NOW

The problem is complicated, we still don't know enough about endometriosis to know whether surgery is helpful for *all* women.

Despite having had nine operations to excise endometriosis, I don't think surgery is the best or only way to manage this disease. Unfortunately it has been necessary for the type of disease I have, which hasn't been controlled by the many hormonal interventions. While surgery has given me some respite and allowed me to get on with my life relatively normally for a long time, my endometriosis keeps coming back and I am left with scar tissue and adhesions that may well be the source of a lot of my pain now, so I am aware of the harm that operating can do. However, even if surgery doesn't resolve your disease, it can provide relief for some time, and for some women not having surgery isn't an option as the disease is causing physical damage and needs to be removed.

Let's make all my surgeries useful!

If you are considering surgery, ask your doctor:
- Why are you recommending surgery rather than hormonal intervention?
- How many people have you treated?
- Are you a specialist in endometriosis, familiar with the complexity of its growth?
- What kind of surgery will you do? Will it be laser or excision? And why?
- What are the risks and complications?
- Where do you believe the disease is? Will you have any other surgeons in attendance if you need e.g., a bowel surgeon or an urologist?
- If you find endometriosis, will you treat it at the time?
- What do you hope the outcome is? No more disease, less pain, better fertility prognosis?

Pack a just-in-case bag

It's likely your surgery will be a day procedure, but always pack an overnight bag and take it with you. You will be asked to go into hospital earlier than the actual operation so it's useful to have distractions.

I packed my hospital bag and in it I put . . .

- **Fat magazines**: full of clothes, make-up and homeware we can't possibly afford. Mindless skimming and pictures provide light relief and really help with the anxiety before surgery.
- **Slippers**: your feet get cold while you wait and just before leaving hospital the nurses will ask you to demonstrate that you can walk a little.
- **Face cream**: that anaesthetic sure dries up your skin.
- **Nice hand cream**: gives you something to do while you wait and it's calming to have a smell you like.
- **A snuggly dressing gown/cardigan**: in case you get a bit cold waiting. Crucially *not* a jumper; they are harder to take off without stretching your core muscles and you need baggy sleeves so you can get them over the cannula needles in the crook of your elbows/hands.
- **Pyjamas**: if you stay over, you might get fed up with the gown and your ass being on show for twenty-four hours. (A good excuse to treat yourself to some new ones too.)
- **A phone charger**: it's amazing how much battery you use while distracting yourself on social media or listening to an audio-book/podcast.
- **A thick sanitary pad**: when you wake up, they will have put a sanitary towel in your paper knickers for any post-op bleeding. It's very thick, like a hunk of bread. It's unlikely you'll have the

energy to change it, but nice to know you can swap it if you want to.

- **An iPad**: download something to distract you ahead of going in (don't forget headphones and remember to pass it to a loved one or put in locker when you go into surgery so it's safe).
- **A book**: disappear into another world for a bit.
- **Your patience**: you may not go in on time or get complete attention from the overstretched medical staff. Any extra stress or anxiety caused by trying to make sense of a situation you can't control will make the pain and experience worse.
- **Your sense of humour**: there's always time for a laugh!

THINGS I KNOW NOW

- Be nice to the nurses. *They* are the ones that come in the middle of the night to help you get to the toilet or give you more pain relief and hold your hand.

- If you are confused about what happened in surgery or what was found, you can ask a nurse on the post-op ward to read your operation notes or ask to see the discharge letter being sent to your GP (you might be given a copy of this anyway).

Tips for leaving hospital
- **Clothes and shoes**: you'll be swollen and uncomfortable so wear loose or stretchy clothing so that nothing is digging into your body and shoes that are easy to slip on so you don't have to bend.

- **Getting home**: you won't be able to drive yourself home because of the anaesthetic and you may need someone to be with you for the first twenty-four hours post-surgery (speak to your doctor or nurse about this). If you don't have someone to drive you, it's worth organising a taxi if possible as you won't feel well enough to use public transport.
- **On the journey home**: use a cushion/pillow/rolled-up jumper between your tummy and the seat belt; it helps reduce the pressure on the incisions. And avoid speed bumps. I learnt this the hard way.

Post-op survival guide

- **Eat good stuff**: you'll feel and heal better, have some vitamins to help your body recover faster (but have some treats too). If you are alone while you recover, try to prepare for this by making meals ahead of the surgery, as you might not feel well enough to stand up and cook.
- **Have distractions**: pre-make a list of TV series and films you can watch when you're zonked and can't make a decision.
- **Try to move a bit**: even if it is just very gently from the sofa to the kitchen, it helps the gas dissipate, gets your bowels moving and reduces restlessness.
- **Don't just stay in your bedroom**: try to keep things as normal as possible and separate day and night.
- **Beware of cabin fever**: go out into the garden or just breathe some fresh air for a few minutes. If you can manage it, get someone to take you out for a little journey in the car. It does wonders for your mood.

Call the doctor/nurse . . .
- if you're worried about the stitches, infection or anything that isn't on the post-op documents.
- if you're constipated, ask for something to soften your stools.
- if you need some more pain relief, it's not weak, it's about *your* body recovering and healing.
- if the painkillers make you nauseous; ask for some anti-nausea tablets.

Here's the stuff I really learnt
- Get some straws or a beaker so you can drink lying down without pulling on abdominal muscles.
- Get an electric heat pad for your lower back while you sit reading/eating/talking/watching TV.
- Drink loads of liquids. Anaesthetic and painkillers make you dehydrated.
- Avoid heavy foods like pasta, pizza, bread. They add to the pressure and create more bloating and constipation.
- Avoid strong laxatives; the urgency and pain will be too much to cope with so use a softener instead, something like Lactulose.
- Ginger or mint tea and sparkling water aid nausea and digestion and also help the gas disperse quicker.
- Having flowers or plants around cheers you up.
- Something to suck on (thank you!). Your mouth can feel weird post-morphine, like you've forgotten how to chew. Boiled sweets are good for this but be warned – I'm now hooked on lemon sherbets!
- Sleep! Don't feel like you can't sleep during the day – this is the best healer.

- Arnica (homeopathy) helps with bruising. Take capsules for a month before and use the tincture in the bath (when incisions are healed a bit).
- Laugh (carefully).

Post-op pain
- Make sure painkillers are easily accessible and you have enough.
- Take painkillers before bed or during the night; you're less likely to wake up in pain.
- If you're taking them in the night, lay them out before you sleep, that way you can set an alarm, take them when you're half-awake and then drift back off.

I got the post-op blues.

It's not uncommon to get a sort of restlessness and profound sadness towards the end of the first week of recovery. It is completely normal to feel a bit miserable and irritable if you're in pain, stuck in the house and on heavy medications, but if you've also had difficult news post-op these feelings can be compounded. However, this can also be a physiological thing too, perhaps even a chemical reaction to the anaesthetic. It's sometimes referred to as post-operative depression and is well documented in medical studies.

- **It will pass**: try to be patient and go easy on yourself.

- **Staying positive and hopeful is really important for recovery**: banish it with distractions, company, comfort and little treats. It might also help to talk to other sufferers who understand what you're going through, in which case online forums might be useful for you during this time (see page 342).

The Endometriosis Wardrobe, Part one: post-op pieces

- **Leggings**: buy one size bigger to allow for swelling. Ideal for when you're leaving the hospital post-surgery, wear them with stretchy tops.
- **Loose dresses, skirts, shirts, t-shirts**: anything comfortable, you don't want tight stuff when you're healing, you need to feel relaxed and unrestricted.
- **Tracksuit bottoms**: comfy but not sluggish, treat yourself to some you really like, it's amazing how what you wear can brighten your mood.
- **Bigger knickers**: ones that don't dig into your hips or tummy. If they have made incisions on the lower abdomen they can be sore and you don't want seams rubbing or adding pressure.
- **Cosy socks/slippers**: feet can get cold when you're not moving much.
- **Flight/compression socks**: they ask you to wear compression socks to reduce the risk of DVT (deep vein thrombosis) while

you're in hospital, but because you don't move much while you recover, they may suggest you continue to wear them for a bit at home (check with nurse). Because they are tight they can get sweaty and itchy so it's good to have another pair (you'll also feel less 'hospitally').

- **Dry shampoo**: not technically a garment, but worth having as it helps you feel mentally better if your hair becomes greasy, but you can't face standing in the shower or washing and drying your hair during the first few days. (Headbands are also great and perk you up a bit.)

Why won't they give me surgery?

Here's where it gets complicated. Some women need to have surgery because the disease is causing organs to stick together so their doctor believes that this is the main cause of pain, and that surgery will help with symptoms and reduce anatomical disease. Other women may be advised that medication, rather than surgery, will be better for their particular disease. It is becoming increasingly common for specialists to begin a hormonal treatment with a working diagnosis of endometriosis based on symptoms or ultrasound scans, without having definitive proof of the presence of endometriosis. I asked Davor Jurkovic, consultant gynaecologist, about this:

Being able to diagnose before surgery is very important. If you make a diagnosis before surgery, everything changes. Although surgery is effective in removing the disease, it does not usually provide a long-term cure. We should look not only at the site of the disease, but we should also assess women's symptoms and try to see whether the location of endometriosis is such that it's a likely to be causing symptoms. If women are routinely given medical treatment after an operation, because the operation does not cure them completely, you have to ask why don't we try medical treatments first?

So in some cases it might be better to avoid invasive surgery if your disease and symptoms can be managed by medication, especially as the usual course of treatment post-op is to have some sort of hormonal treatment anyway. I spoke to my own Dr B about this:

> If a patient's pain can be controlled on medication it is best to avoid a laparoscopy. Surgery is only warranted when pain is not controlled on medication, if fertility is an issue, if the volume of disease is increasing (for example, an endometrioma – a cyst – is enlarging on scan), or when women simply want a diagnosis.

It's not unusual to prefer the idea of surgery to taking hormonal treatments but many women find that the milder hormonal intervention, such as the pill or coil are very beneficial and the side effects manageable, we'll go into this more in the next chapter. Such things helped me with the symptoms for many years in between surgeries. If your specific disease isn't affecting you anatomically (i.e. sticking organs together) it might be worth pursuing hormone treatment over surgery for now.

The symptoms have got worse, it must be everywhere now surely?

If the pain comes back or continues after a surgery, one is inclined to think it must be because there is new disease. Doctors may push back on this idea if they believe the source of the pain is to do with nerves and inflammation rather than the disease itself. I spoke to Katy Vincent, a consultant gynaecologist and pelvic-pain specialist:

> I try to avoid repeating surgeries until we have done everything else because surgery has associated risks and there can be huge disappointment if you don't find anything. If you still have a neuropathic component, or muscular spasms in your pelvis, you are not going to get better from the surgery so it is a waste of time. Let's first try other things, for example try to damp down your neuropathic component and sort your pelvic floor.

If a doctor suggests medication rather than further surgery you might well feel exasperated. It's not that women with endometriosis are inherently surgery-happy, we just want the pain to end. Our cultural perception around disease and illness also has a part to play here: we are conditioned to think that surgical removal is likely to be a better option than taking some pills. This isn't surprising. If you're told that you have a disease that sticks organs together, is the cause of your pain and may have an effect on your fertility, I think everyone would say: 'You're not proposing we leave it in there are you?' But the problem is, we still don't know enough about it and no one can be sure that it is the disease itself that's causing the pain, so cutting it out might make no difference at all for some. I asked Dr B:

> I think that you have to be very careful to avoid simply resorting to more surgery. If it has worked well in the past and a woman wants a further laparoscopy then it would be reasonable.

However, it is important to be realistic about the chances of improving symptoms, especially if surgery has not been of particular benefit in the past. In many cases if medication controls symptoms, surgery can be avoided or at the very least postponed.

And Davor Jurkovic added:

I see women who have spent years desperate to find a spot of endometriosis but it's not there. So, I try to get them to see that endometriosis is only one of the causes of pelvic pain. The endometriosis causes pelvic pain but not every part of the disease causes pain. There are also many women with severe endometriosis who are free of any pain. It puts into focus this difficult question: if you operate on the endometriosis success-fully and the woman is still unwell, could it be something other than endometriosis causing the pain? I see a lot of people who suffer with pain without visible disease and they tend to blame it on the doctors not being successful in finding endometriosis. We have not made this shift yet from focusing on abnormal anatomy to women's individual experiences of pain.

It's hard to accept that the pain might not be caused by the endo-metriosis itself and it's even harder not to imagine an angry, mutating, sticky disease and to quieten all the fears we have about what will happen if it's left untreated. But this is why awareness and understanding is so important; not everyone's disease is like this. It's a complex condition, so it's vital the treatment of it is tailored to your disease and what's best for your life and plans.

> **THINGS I KNOW NOW**
>
> If your specialist is recommending other medical treatments ask why they are reluctant to do surgery in your case. Having a thorough understanding of your treatment plan is very important as it reduces anxiety and gives you more control.

Hysterectomy

Every endometriosis specialist I've spoken to told me this should be a last resort, no one should recommend it as a 'quick' solution. This is an irreversible procedure, with life-altering consequences. It's major surgery and a big decision. It needs consideration and a thorough understanding of what will happen afterwards. Depending on your disease, a hysterectomy may not resolve your pain. It also comes with side effects. It's more complicated than 'just taking it all out'.

Here's why:

- You will be instantly menopausal.
- It won't *definitely* stop the growth; you may still have endometrial deposits.
- It doesn't work for everyone.
- The pain might not be disease related now; it could be nerve or tissue damage in the wider peritoneum.
- The lack of natural oestrogen can have an effect on other parts of your body: bones, bladder, bowel, thyroid, sexual function.

For some women, intolerable physical pain versus the emotional pain of never bearing children become their 'choices' and as drastic as it may seem, some decide to have a hysterectomy in the hope it will give them respite. For the women I've spoken to, this was a difficult and life-changing decision, with emotional and physical ramifications, but they did get relief from symptoms for some time, although usually it hasn't been a cure for them (see the interviews on pages 303–336).

For this to be an effective treatment depends hugely on the type of disease *you* have, *your* body's response and the skill of the surgeon; all endometrial deposits in the peritoneal cavity must be removed. Keep talking to your doctor about it if this is something you are considering or is being suggested as a treatment. Make sure you are *fully informed* before doing it.

9

Hormone treatment

It's hard for people who don't have endometriosis to grasp the lengths we go to, and the risks and suffering we endure, to get control of this disease and live something resembling a normal life. Frightening treatments are often suggested by doctors with such nonchalance one would have thought they were listing the types of coffee available on a menu. Even if you really don't want to have the treatment being offered, you might also feel you don't have a choice, that you have to try one or more of them to get the disease and symptoms under control.

There is no treatment or drug designed specifically for endometriosis even though 200 million women worldwide are known to be suffering. What's even crazier to me is that the treatment options haven't changed in the fifteen years since I was diagnosed. The researchers at the Oxford Endometriosis CaRe Centre told me that there is potential for precision medicine, a drug specially designed for endometriosis, but this is reliant on further research and that requires a vast increase in funding to make it possible. So, for now, endometriosis borrows medications from other parts of medicine, ones designed for general neuropathic pain, hormonal drugs, sometimes ones originally meant to treat cancer or seizures. Your doctor may suggest managing your disease and symptoms through hormone treatments, such as the pill, Mirena coil or hormonal injections. These options provide contraception but also help regulate your cycle and minimise or stop heavy, regular bleeding. There are also other stronger treatments such as GnRH, which create a temporary pseudo-menopause, but as these are more invasive drugs they should be tried after other treatments haven't been successful.

The medication effect

Because the medications aren't tailored to suit our individual bodies, we take the same tablets or have the same injections whether we're a size eight or eighteen, and it's probable we're taking a much larger dose of something than we need for the effects. For example, I feel pretty ropey the day after I have a lot of sugar, and if I consumed a lot of sugar every day I would feel increasingly awful and pretty unwell all the time. Gradually this would become the norm and I would get used to trying to live in that level of discomfort. This is exactly how I feel on hormones.

Now then mardy bum

For most women our natural cycle and hormones affect mood; PMS can make us irritable and miserable. But if you have endometriosis then you're likely to have large doses of synthetic hormones and pain medications in your system. It's no wonder we sometimes feel crazy, moody, anxious or depressed. The effect of hormone treatments on mood can make it hard to distinguish between what your *real* response to the situation is, and what is created or magnified by the medications The problem is, hormonal treatments are the only thing that doctors have to offer to manage the symptoms at the moment (apart from surgery), and for some women access to surgery is not possible, so hormonal treatments are the only option.

THINGS I KNOW NOW

Hormones are a bitch.

- It may take a few months for your body to get used to a treatment, but if the effects are unmanageable go back to your doctor.

- The artificial hormones might make you feel things more intensely, it's important to recognise this. There is hope that because these emotions aren't 'real' it's not what you actually feel so it will pass and get easier.

- How do you not feel crazy in the meantime? Tracking your cycle can help you to recognise cyclical emotions.

- Treatments and their side effects are not universal in their efficacy or tolerability; one drug may work well for one woman but be useless for another. It's often a case of trial and error to find the best one for you.

- It can take several months for your natural cycle to resume when you stop taking hormonal treatments but if you're worried, see your doctor.

We are not a guinea pig

Synthetic hormones are used by millions of women across the globe for contraception, to regulate menstruation and to avoid heavy and messy periods, but also to manage issues like acne and PMS, and reproductive conditions like endometriosis, polycystic ovaries (PCOs) and fibroids. I don't want to diminish the huge importance that access to birth control brings to women's lives. It grants us the autonomy and freedom to manage our bodies, reproduction and sexual activity, but these drugs also come with risks and side effects that many women cannot or do not wish to tolerate. Women taking these medications often experience headaches, mood swings, weight gain, nausea, never-ending periods, depression, acne, muscle weakness or aching, changes to hair and skin. Some women I know have had migraines or visual disturbance, sleep issues or sudden onset anger. While the pills themselves are small, the effect on our systems can be massive, but this is the compromise we often make in order to have control of our bodies and lives.

Interestingly, research trials for a 'male pill' or hormonal injection have invariably come to a halt when participants complain of adverse and intolerable side effects such as mood swings, depression and acne. The gender bias here is stark: the trials stop because men feel comfortable saying the effects are unacceptable, that they couldn't be expected to endure them and, most of all, they were listened to. Yet *women* have been handling these effects for decades now, simply assuming this is the deal: in order to have autonomy we have to be prepared to accept the side effects.

Women with endometriosis sometimes have to take high doses or a combination of medications to manage their disease and the effects can be disruptive and sometimes even intolerable. But it can be a hard 'choice' between trying to manage your symptoms without treatment and taking hormonal medications to suppress the symptoms but dealing with their side effects. Indeed, for many women birth control is the only option available to manage endometriosis, because their insurance or health system doesn't allow them access to surgery, whether it's necessary in their case or not. In some parts of the world women won't have access to *any* of these medical treatments and they have to struggle on without any medical support at all.

You've done it all!

I have been medicated in some form since I was seventeen, swapping and changing hormone and pain medications, and I haven't been comfortable in my body for most of that time. In order to suppress or remove the disease we undergo some pretty unpleasant things. If you become desperate and the symptoms are unmanageable, it is not unusual to try anything that might help, even if it seems drastic. Since I was diagnosed I've had two pseudo-menopauses and lots of other treatments, but I hardly talked about the effects on the rest of my body and my mental health. I just tried to get on with it, hoping they would work. I've found it hard to find much support or guidance on how to manage the effects of the stronger hormone medications, but I think it helps if we're honest about what it's *really* like, so we don't feel so alone. I haven't included my experiences to frighten you, more in hope that by having an insight into particular treatments it might help you if you're going through something similar.

GnRH (age 20)

Just before my twentieth birthday I had my fourth surgery and Dr B suggested I begin a year-long pseudo-menopause treatment called GnRH to suppress the rapid growth of the disease. I'm at university in Sussex so I've just been to the campus nurse to have an injection in my arse cheek. The needle squeezed in a thick gel that sits in my system, releasing as the month goes on. It spreads slowly and my body resists it. My cheek is so sore I have to lean on the other one when I sit or sleep. For once I'm grateful I have enough 'cushion' in my bottom. I spend the next few days binge-watching *Desperate Housewives* and sleeping. Hopefully it won't hurt as much next month, maybe I'll even start to feel better, that would be nice.

* * *

I'm about five months in and despite taking HRT, and all the calcium and magnesium I can get my hands on, I'm nauseous and achy. I have hot flushes and night sweats and I've gained a couple of stone. It's like having flu all the time, I just can't seem to get going. I'm in my first year at university but I'm missing it all. I have become a recluse, barely leaving my flat. I'm anxious and fear people can see I'm ill. My eyes dart around the room and I feel panic when I'm invited to do something. A jaunt out in Brighton? Staying up all night at a party? I feel timid and nervous, and worried about what my body might do. I don't tell anyone what is going on. I don't want to be weird. I stop going to lectures altogether. I can't get up in time, even the idea of hauling my limbs out of bed and down to the hall is enough to make me drag the duvet over my head and go back to sleep. My boyfriend comes to stay and I have all sorts of nice things planned but when he gets here I'm too exhausted, so we have some quiet meals in the communal kitchen and try to sleep in a single bed together. It's miserable.

* * *

We eventually break up. He's young and hasn't signed up for this. I was supposed to be a carefree twenty-year-old, not a woman in her fifties. I leave this university at the end of the first year, it's too hard to be this far away from home and so ill. I start at Manchester instead. I'm reminded of the words often attributed to Marilyn Monroe: 'Sometimes good things fall apart, so that better things can fall together.' She's right, this is one of the best decisions I've made, and I made it because of the disease. So occasionally it does something useful. Oh, and I get a new boyfriend.

* * *

I've made it to a year on this drug and I'm relieved when Dr B says I can come off it. It takes a couple of months but I begin to feel like myself again. My body goes back to normal with a few symptoms left over: my skin is a bit drier and I get the occasional hot flush. I start to take the pill back to back again in three-month intervals, so I only have four periods a year, and the side effects now feel like nothing compared to GnRH.

* * *

This treatment might have helped to suppress the disease somewhat because I didn't have another operation for just over two years. However, the symptoms became pretty unmanageable again after around fifteen months, so for symptom control I don't think it was worth it. Ten years later, before I embarked on another drastic treatment, I had a bone scan to see if the GnRH had had any affect on my bone density. It had.

How do you decide on a treatment

If you have been suffering for a long time (with or without a diagnosis) you become so used to being bustled in and out of appointments, overwhelmed and exhausted by it all, and you can end up agreeing to things you don't understand, or don't want to do. The pressure to make a quick decision means even *we* forget that we have lives to go back to and the treatments might have an impact on them.

Take some time to consider the options and their implications, there's no rush.

Oestrogen (age 30)

I've just had my eighth surgery and my thirtieth birthday. DR B has suggested a drastic treatment, a drug called anastrozole, which blocks the creation of oestrogen. It is actually licensed for breast cancer and is usually prescribed for post-menopausal women after chemotherapy. It sounds terrifying, but I feel pressure to try something because I can't keep having surgery this regularly. Dr B is cautious but there aren't many options left now. I don't understand endometriosis; it makes no sense. It's like the disease version of a worm: you cut its head off but it just grows back. In the car I allow myself the length of a Bob Dylan song to lose my shit, digest the information and create a plan. Then I drive home intent on researching my options.

* * *

The more I read about this treatment the more I'm reluctant to do it. I trust Dr B, but even he has said this will be grim and that I should seek advice from other specialists. I get second and third opinions. All agree it's pretty extreme but are stumped when I ask for alternatives. My 'choices' are limited: an aggressive treatment or hysterectomy. I agree to try it. The plan is to take anastrozole and the pill (to protect my bones) and a Mirena coil; so, my body thinks it is post-menopausal and pregnant all at once? Talk about a hormonal tug of war! My GP thinks it's too radical so refuses to prescribe it, so I have the added bonus of paying for a treatment that is likely to make me feel very poorly.

* * *

The side effects are supposed to be similar to GnRH but that turns out to have been a bed of roses by comparison. Menopause is a slower, natural process and (usually) happens at the right time in a woman's reproductive life. This artificial menopause happens very quickly to a body that, at thirty years old, isn't expecting it. I start to notice the effects overnight. It turns out you need oestrogen for quite a lot of stuff. Without it I have blurred vision, aching bones and sore teeth and jaw. I gain a couple of stone. My skin is dry and sore. My hair is thin, greasy and starts to fall out. My joints hurt, I have no strength in my muscles and I'm nauseous and swollen all the time. Otherwise I'm fine.

* * *

I have to sit down to put my socks on and take breaks drying my hair because the dryer is too heavy. I break things, tip drinks over my computer and walk into stuff. I pour milk into the cafetière (middle-class problems) and turn up to places on the wrong day or not at all. My sex drive is so low and I'm so unbothered about it all, I'm considering putting my vibrator on Freecycle. Every bag has a packet of tissues in it to dab the excessive sweat. There's no logic to it. I drip making a cup of tea – hardly a Jane Fonda workout! Gone are the days when I can take a small purse out with me, I have so many tranklements and tablets, I need a large handbag and people say annoying things like 'Moving in are we?'

* * *

I've no appetite, I feel bilious all the time, like I'm on a boat, and I get a burning sensation when I eat. My morning walk to the train station involves walking through south London

– not a place to be breathing deeply if you're feeling queasy. The smells meld together: fishmongers and frying bacon, coffee and drains, heavy petrol and hot plastic fill the air amid the cannabis and cigarette smoke, the streets are made of urine and last night's vomit.

* * *

I feel very low and lonely. I try to remember it isn't real but this anxiety is new, I don't want to go out. I find big groups of people overwhelming. Even the *idea* of a party fills me with dread. I've begun to lose all my joy and I'm too tired to notice the little things that would usually make me laugh. I've only told close friends and family and my work don't know. I'm determined that I can handle this on my own, that it will be worth it if it's finally the fix we've been searching for, but it's getting harder to hide it from people, especially in front of the boy I had a thing with and now have to see every day. My hairdresser Natalie has done amazing things to cover up the bald patches at the front of my hair. I've bought comfortable, floaty clothes and put the ones that don't fit in a box under the bed so I feel less gloomy when I open the wardrobe.

* * *

This isn't endometriosis any more, it isn't cyclical, it is all day, every day. After two months I ask if I can come off it. Dr B tells me it would be good if I could make it to three months (the length of time it takes for a drug to really kick into your system). The side effects might settle. It feels like a waste of time to have gone through all this for nothing. Maybe it *will* get easier? Or I'll get used to it.

* * *

Online I can't find anyone who has taken anastrozole for endometriosis. I commit the cardinal sin of googling it and end up on the cancer sites. I find a testimonial from a woman whose teeth fell out when she stopped taking it. I ring my mum, who tells me to stop reading and then I call the dentist and vow to be vigilant about my calcium intake. At the theatre that night I tell my friend Trevor and he cries with laughter, while also apologising because it isn't funny at all. I start to sing 'All I Want for Christmas is My Two Front Teeth'. I am consoled by the idea that there is always time for a laugh, but as I sing I'm very aware that my teeth hurt.

* * *

It occurs to me that these treatments are like a try-before-you-buy scheme. When the real menopause comes round I will have already been through it twice. I'm going to smash those symptoms out of the park – they'll be a walk in the park. I'll be a menopause guru and all the women I love will come for advice and I'll be able to help because I've been here before. I'll be a connoisseur of the hot flush, the aching bones and the hair tricks. Not much help now, but a comfort to think it might be useful for the future.

* * *

Anastrozole was supposed to stop the disease growing, but it was also stopping me from doing much else. I began to rely heavily on a concoction of painkillers to keep my job and some semblance of a life. I managed six months and then begged Dr B to let me come off it. When I did my body ground to a complete halt. I didn't leave the house for six weeks. This is by far the worst drug I have ever experienced and the most poorly I have ever been in my life. And I had to have surgery a year later anyway – damn this disease!

THINGS I KNOW NOW

How to survive horrible hormone treatments.

- Drink lots of water; it flushes your system, but hydration also helps with the nausea, fainting, dry skin and mouth.

- Eye drops; great for dry or tired eyes that sometimes come with meds.

- Ginger and turmeric for inflammation and joint ache.

- High-strength vitamins help support your system.

- Mint tea and apple juice are soothing.

- Anti-nausea tablets from your doctor.

- If you're nauseous or have no appetite, a temporary solution is to get a blender so you still get the vital nutrients your body needs under stress.

- Arnica gel for your hands and feet; put the gel on at night though because it's a bit sticky and peels off like PVA glue.

- Heat (bags, bottles, electric blankets, you name it).

- Ring your friends; keep doing stuff even if they just come to chill out with you.

- Don't lie in a lump in bed unless you really have to, at least go and lump it on the sofa and watch something nice.

When the drugs don't work

If you've tried several treatments that haven't worked to suppress your disease or manage your symptoms you can begin to have low expectations of what doctors can offer and it can make you cautious of trying anything else. If you've also experienced devastating physical and mental side effects but the treatment still hasn't worked, it can make you feel jaded and despondent, worried that you'll never find anything that will help.

THINGS I KNOW NOW

- Please don't give up. Talk to your specialist about what they can do to help manage your disease and what else you might be able to try.

- There are other ways to alleviate symptoms. Keep reading . . .

However mild the doctors tell me the hormones are, my body doesn't like them, it's like it resists them somehow and the more drastic hormone therapies haven't worked for me either. It's very confusing when the things that ought to suppress periods and oestrogen aren't working for us but we don't know why. I asked Professor Krina Zondervan about this and I learnt something new:

> The endometriosis tissue itself produces oestrogen. Therefore endometrial deposits generate their own hormonal feedback and create their own hormonal micro-environment. This means that whilst they are still susceptible to your internal hormonal changes, on top of that they have got their own 'supply' as well. This may also explain why, and particularly in women who have had endometriosis for a long time, pain is not 'just' bad with periods or sex but can become fairly constant. Not just cyclical, you can have a lot of symptoms a lot of the time. Whilst this may be one reason for persistent pain, the short answer is not that satisfying, which is to say we don't really know yet why some women experience the pain they do and others don't, and why hormone treatments work for some but not for others.

For some women hormone therapies do seem to temper the disease, for others they don't respond and we need to research that more to understand why.

This might explain why I haven't been able to find an effective or tolerable hormonal treatment because my disease is atypical, so the medical management for me is a combination of low-impact hormonal intervention, pain management and surgery as and when I need it.

10

Talking to doctors

I've been very lucky that I've had the same endometriosis doctor since I was diagnosed, it is one of the things that has kept me sane. Over the years we have built a strong, supportive relationship. I trust him, his knowledge and his advice. Dr B's compassion, honesty and determination to help me live my life as pain- and symptom-free as possible and his belief in me as a person (not just a patient) has been vital. At no point has he been flippant, dismissive or made me feel like anything is my fault. It doesn't take a lot to be like this. It doesn't make the appointment longer, or mean I'm constantly asking for his help. His clarity actually means I see him less. I wish for every woman with endometriosis to have a Dr B of their own.

THINGS I KNOW NOW

- Consistency is important especially with an inconsistent, long term and complex disease; it builds trust, understanding and more personalised care.

> • It's possible that you may have to see numerous doctors and specialists, as well as alternative therapists, but try to build a team where possible; a knowledgeable GP and endometriosis specialist are crucial long-term.

Despite this support, I've still had more gynaecologists than hot dinners. I know how hard it can be to talk to doctors and get what you need from the appointment, especially if they are intimidating, dismissive or irritated that you're back again asking for help.

Help with talking to doctors

We often have to see a different doctor and repeat our whole history all over again, trying to remember the important medical bits and omitting the days lost, sleepless nights, the pain so bad you cry involuntarily and moan into a pillow. We get very good at reeling off a succinct symptom list that's detached from the reality of living with this condition. We give short, relevant answers like we're dropping a car off for an MOT. If you haven't got to this point yet or you're still seeking a diagnosis or a more manageable treatment plan, here are some tips to help you get the most out of the appointment:

- **Do some research**: learn about the various options so you know which one you're more likely to want to try, and what concerns you about them.
- **Think about what you want to ask**: make a short list of questions beforehand so you don't forget anything.

- **Think about the outcome**: what do you want to happen? Referrals? Further tests? Surgery? A clearer understanding? It guides the appointment, gives you some control and makes it harder for the doctor to dismiss you.
- **Don't be afraid to ask for referrals**: to see different doctors – pain specialists, physiotherapists and endocrinologists.

THINGS I KNOW NOW

- Talk to your doctor about your options, then go home and think about it.

- Do some more research, talk to your loved ones and ask their advice before you commit. You only have one body.

Don't go alone

When I was first diagnosed I felt very strongly that I wanted to be in the appointments alone; that this was the best way for me to process the information. I could work out what I felt without being concerned about anyone else's feelings. In retrospect this wasn't a great idea. There were often times I wished I had taken someone with me, even if they just sat in the waiting room. I also came to realise that I'd have to explain it all over again anyway, which was exhausting. More recently, having someone with me has been a huge consolation. It's surprising how you can forget what is being said if it's distressing or the doctor speaks very fast. You're allowed to say, 'This is difficult and I need some support'. Think about who would be the most useful for you in this situation: a friend, parent, partner? Depending on your preference, they can be vocal advocates or just take notes so you have them for reference later on.

Appointments with specialists

Because it is a multifaceted condition there may be lots of elements to talk about: pain relief, symptom control, treatment of the disease.

- Make sure they explain the treatment plan, the diagnosis and prognosis and your choices.
- The plan should take into account your life, work, relationships, age, fertility.
- Ask questions: what are the outcomes? Possible risks and side effects? It helps to be aware of what to expect.
- Don't be afraid to tell them if you want to change the plan or that you don't understand.
- Is there anything *you* can do to help manage symptoms? Physiotherapy, pain-management techniques? If they don't know, ask who might.

Letters (age 17–33)

I've seen so many doctors I've stopped counting, my private parts are all over the country (and not in a good way). One of the downsides of having so many doctors is the mountain of paperwork I end up with. Now I have to do filing for my uterus too. I get copies of the consultant letters to my GP, but because they're written from doctor to doctor they're full of medical terminology and things can appear much less serious on paper than they had led me to believe in the appointment. It's another layer of dismissal when I read phrases like 'she denies she experiences this' or 'to a mild degree'. The language is so detached, as though they are describing a vessel, not a person. 'I saw this young lady in my clinic today' – you had your hand in my vagina. I think you might be able to use my name! But the most unbearable moment is when a letter says, 'In view of normal investigations I have not organised any further follow-up.' The despair is overwhelming when you realise that you're going to have to embark on *more* research and find *another* person who might be able to help. It's like a game of snakes and ladders: you think you're progressing and then you slip down a snake and have to start all over again.

THINGS I KNOW NOW

- **Try to get copies of your notes, letters, scans, operation reports**: having all the information when you go to see different doctors saves time and energy and reduces the chance of repeated tests and dismissal.

- **Be nice to the secretaries**: (you should be anyway) but they have the ability to change appointments, get hold of the doctors urgently, send you medical documents.

Don't be intimidated

If doctors talk in medical language or suggest your case isn't serious, it can make you feel like you're wasting their time and I know the fear of being perceived as defiant or difficult when you keep asking questions. It's made harder because you have to talk about the most private parts of your body and life, so it's not surprising that we sometimes cower in the clinics of specialists and daren't mention our true concerns. My strategy to handle this is to think of other experts I wouldn't be intimidated by; if this was my car and I was talking to a mechanic I wouldn't see it as hassling them to explain what work needs doing and why is the bill is that amount? If my hairdresser said something about my hair but didn't explain it properly before they started hacking away I'd be rightly nervous and probably ask for clarity. Why should doctors be any different?

WIWIS (age 30)

I once paid a fortune to see a head honcho for a second opinion. He told me: 'I'm a technician, I cut it out.' (He literally cuts and runs.) 'I have no real knowledge or interest in why the disease grows, I'm the practical one, you need to speak to a medical, more bookish one for that.'

Why wasn't he curious about why a disease he has dedicated his entire medical career to mutates and grows? Why didn't he want to learn? Why did he bother to do it at *all* when we know surgery isn't a fix anyway? His wanton limiting of knowledge was infuriating and arrogant. I didn't know doctors could specify their area of interest in such a restrictive way. I wish the world were like this for all of us; I like to eat all the food but I don't like the washing-up, I leave that to someone else. I like to drink copious amounts of champagne but I have no interest in having a hangover, someone else can have that.

I often think of the best thing to say after the fact, which is not much help as a person but good for a writer. I call these WIWIS (what I wish I'd said), which makes me smile because it's jaunty and short, and because it sounds like wee-wees. Laughing at something gives me a bit of control back; I become the puppeteer not the puppet. WIWIS is what I long to be able to say: 'I'm a specialist in endometriosis but I don't care much for having it myself so I'm not going to bother, thanks all the same, give it to someone else.' But really WIWIS to *that* doctor is: 'Gosh what a limited and dismal approach you have. Apologies that my credit card bounced when you charged me to do nothing and refer me on. I like to spend money, I'm the practical one, I don't worry about where it comes from, you'll want to speak to the more bookish people at the bank for that.'

We don't need surgery-focused doctors. We need the doctors who make the life-changing decisions about us to be informed, curious, kind and interested. I want them to be rehearsed in all aspects of the disease. The decisions I have to make are not just whether I do or don't have children. The treatments can have life-altering implications too: weight gain, muscles aching, bones breaking, whether I can ride a bike, dance, have sex.

THINGS I KNOW NOW

Demand that they consider *you* as a person not just as a list of symptoms to be dealt with. A good doctor will ask about your life and plans and tailor the treatment plan to you.

If this were happening to your parent or your child you would push hard for answers. You need to treat yourself like that.

Managing expectations

What doctors can offer may be frustrating and slow, they are trying their best with limited medical treatments, but you may need to push for more support and recognise that you can do things to help manage the symptoms too (more on that in a bit). With the current financial constraints on the health system it can be difficult to offer good, consistent management for long-term illness and unfortunately endometriosis falls into this category. However, your doctor should see the person in front of them and approach with kindness and understanding. If they can't cure it, they should at least try to help us to *live* with it. If you feel that you are not being heard or don't trust your doctor, walk away and find another one.

The Endometriosis Manual

We are not always perfect patients, we can be difficult and angry, we can exacerbate the symptoms by our behaviour and choices, by resisting the realities of the disease.

But there isn't a manual for living with endometriosis, often we are just trying to get to grips with it. We're not all medically trained, we don't know if there are things we should or shouldn't be worrying about. This is new territory. Don't let anyone diminish your coping strategies or concerns.

It takes a lot to laugh; it takes a dismissive doctor to cry

If we are told often enough that our symptoms or pain are normal or all in our head, that it's because we eat too much pasta or are overstressed and we should maybe consider mindfulness, we'll stop asking for help. It's frustrating and despairing and can feel like you're wasting your time. Access to specialists may not be readily available, but it would help women significantly if the medical community understood endometriosis better. Even after the coveted diagnosis, I've still experienced dismissal from doctors and shockingly met many that haven't even heard of it or who have such a limited understanding (or misunderstanding) of it I might as well have stayed at home and self-medicated. It's likely that you have become (because you've had to become) more of an expert than the experts themselves and it can be incredibly frustrating when you are given wrong, confusing or contradictory information.

I'm routinely told the disease is cured now I've had surgery, that having a baby or a hysterectomy will cure it, that I'm hypersensitive, that it can't be that bad or I just have to accept it. It can be hard to deal with doctors that dismiss our experience, that rush and belittle us and don't understand the far-reaching effects this condition can have on our lives. Trying to communicate with these particular doctors is challenging. They don't like it if you start telling them what you need, it can be mistaken for being difficult or rude. The problem is, when you live with endometriosis you *know* your body and it's hard to remain calm and reasonable when the people who are supposed to be helping you aren't.

Doctors are not gods, they make mistakes sometimes and they don't always have the answers. A good doctor will recognise if they haven't got the expertise and refer you to someone who does or talk to you about treatments not cures. But some have too big an ego to let you know that they can't help and they don't like it if you become an expert patient asking lots of questions, because it magnifies their inadequacies. That's when they get defensive and make you feel small and stupid.

THINGS I KNOW NOW

How to handle dismissal

- **Remember this is one person**: they don't get to decide what happens after you leave that room.

- **Ring someone you love**: cry, laugh, get angry, despair, but it's always better to talk rather than keep it inside.

- **Try to remain optimistic**: approach each doctor/nurse with a fresh mind, reserve judgement, recognise them on their own merit and give them the benefit of the doubt. They might be the one that can help you this time.

- **Remember the other women**: I feel empowered, stronger and less alone if I think of all the other women before and after me that have been in the same situation.

- **Walk away**: you don't have to stay or do what they say.

The E-Team

One of the biggest difficulties I have faced when trying to manage endometriosis is that there doesn't seem to be much joined-up thinking. I see one doctor for the endometriosis and one for the pain, another prescribes the medication and another advises on hormones and fertility. No one is looking at the whole picture – just their little bit of it – and it's a completely illogical way to work, especially with something that affects each woman so differently.

Endometriosis is a complex condition that may require support from multiple practitioners at different times but it's often up to the patient to link up all the information. Trying to create your own team of people is exhausting (and sometimes expensive) but it can also result in trying several treatments all at once, which makes it hard to know what is working or indeed whether some of the symptoms might even be being caused by one treatment interacting badly with another, e.g. hormones with painkillers.

If the pain issues are connected to the disease and surgeries, we need our GP and pain doctors to have a good understanding of the intricacies of endometriosis *and* pelvic pain, so they can help us to manage it better. But if their awareness of the condition is limited or inaccurate, then it's likely we'll go home feeling frustrated and unsupported, or worse, given unnecessary or the wrong kind of treatment.

The current medical approach is to treat endometriosis as though it's an 'acute' not a 'chronic' condition, reacting to the urgent issue rather than providing long-term support to live with it. But in complex and persistent cases of endometriosis where the symptoms change or become unmanageable, I believe that much of the distress and confusion that we experience could be avoided or at least reduced by a multidisciplinary, long-term team approach. The E-Team. Sadly due to the current limitations on the health-care system, this is not standard practice, and many women find there is little consistency of care nor a plan in place if symptoms worsen, so we seek help from multiple sources, often privately, in order to cope, or find ourselves in A&E because there is no 'urgent' support available to us.

What would this E-Team look like?
- On diagnosis women would be assigned to a specialist clinical team: an informed GP, an endometriosis consultant and/or surgeon, a nurse specialist, a physiotherapist, a psychotherapist and a nutritionist.
- If the pain becomes more problematic, we would have access to a pelvic-pain specialist; if we have fertility issues, we would be able to see a fertility expert (who understands endometriosis).

Most women wouldn't need to access this level of support for the majority of the time, some may never need it, or only need it for a short time, or only need parts of it, but this support ought to be available if we are taking this condition as seriously as it should be taken.

How else would it help?

- Case histories could be regularly updated and available on a database accessible to the team (with permission, this could also work as a research tool, helping to increase understanding of the condition).
- It would be less stressful for the patient (did anyone remember that stress makes all the symptoms worse?) who currently has to access help from scratch each time the symptoms flare up and they need support; e.g. having to go to A&E with pain or issues with cysts.
- Long term it would reduce strain on the health system; primary care might be expensive to develop initially, but early intervention is far cheaper than responding to health conditions in an emergency or trying to reverse the effects of something that has been left untreated for some time, particularly with regards to persistent pain.

It may sound like an ambitious proposal but endometriosis is a complicated disease that requires a multidisciplinary approach. If the treatment options are limited the very least that should be offered is a support system to help women *live* with it. Having a dedicated clinical team is not such a radical suggestion either; such systems already exist for other long-term medical issues. Indeed, BSGE centres offer something similar, but there are still too few of them in the UK and many GPs are not as aware of their work as they need to be given the number of women who are suffering.

I believe this structured support would not only reduce unnecessary surgeries, tests, misdiagnoses and reliance on heavy and addictive pain medication, but it would be hugely beneficial for many women who could avoid much of the misery that comes with having to cobble together their own support network and team.

11
Other ways to manage symptoms

Isn't there a pamphlet or something?

I have often felt very alone trying to cope and actually *live* with endometriosis as though it was entirely down to me to sort it out. I wanted someone to tell me how to handle all this stuff, how was I supposed to just know? So in this chapter I'm going to share with you what I have learnt and what coping strategies I have developed over the years through a combination of trial and error, practice and visiting a lot of clever people. I have cherry-picked my brain and while this chapter is a bit bigger than a pamphlet, I hope it helps.

THINGS I KNOW NOW

- Develop coping strategies that work for you, ones you can rely on to get you through, even on the bad days.

- Don't give up; there is relief, even if there isn't a fix.

- Become educated and ask lots of questions; it's *your* body.

- There are many ways to manage it, not all of them are invasive or medical.

- Endometriosis doesn't define you but it's important to recognise that it can sometimes have a huge impact on your life, even if it's only a few days a month, and these effects can be both physical and psychological.

- Consider the effects on your mental and emotional health. I didn't really think about the implications of living with a long-term, painful condition until I had to.

- You need a strong support network and a crack medical team.

- Try to be realistic about your capabilities and limitations; this will help you avoid crashes, increased symptoms and pain 'spikes'.

- Don't beat yourself up for the botches you're making to get through it.

- Be gentle and patient with your body, it's managing a challenging condition. Try not to get too angry with it or begin to hate it (more on that later.)

Is this all you have to offer?

I became used to being in major discomfort and felt guilty for taking up time asking for help for something that couldn't be fixed. But I kept going back, knowing that hormones or surgery were the only options, yet hoping there might be *something* the doctors could do. Isn't the definition of madness to keep doing the same thing expecting a different outcome? That's me then. I'm mad. But I just wanted to get on with my life with the least amount of medication and surgery as possible and to not have to be so conscious of my body.

Nothing is more exasperating than when a doctor looks at you blankly as though you're expecting too much when you ask for better options than those they are offering. I could accept the diagnosis, I could accept the disappointment that came with trying things that didn't work and I knew by now that it was too much to ask for no side effects at *all*, but I couldn't understand why everyone was content with such bad options to manage this disease. I didn't want a second or third opinion; I wanted a different one. I wanted someone to see me as a *person*, not just a patient and help me to *live* with endometriosis.

Going private

I live in the UK where we have the NHS (National Health Service), a state health system that is paid for by our taxes. As my dad says, 'It's like an insurance policy we hope we don't have to use.' Unlike private medical systems, the NHS has no hidden extra costs, excesses or stoppage of treatment if you can't afford it. No matter what you earn you will have healthcare. It is a world-class service that has looked after me, all the people I love, will love and have loved, it has brought my nieces and nephews into the world and cared for my loved ones when they are sick, frightened and dying. I am extremely lucky to have been born in a country that has this service, especially because I have endometriosis. All of my nine surgeries have been done under the NHS and I have received extraordinary care and support from many doctors and nurses.

But even this system has limitations, particularly when it comes to complicated and long-term illness, which means I often have to supplement my treatments with private support. Over the years I have spent thousands of pounds on alternative therapies, specialists and various diagnostic tests to manage my symptoms. I know how lucky I am to be able to do this and that not everyone can afford to access extra paid support, but I want to share with you some tips on how to navigate *these* private parts if, and when, you use them.

So why go private?

You may want to pay to get quicker tests or access a specific treatment that is not available through the NHS. You may need to see a psychologist, or a pelvic-pain specialist more urgently, or perhaps the support being offered is for a limited number of sessions and you need more. However, it is important to recognise the false impression that private health care is automatically superior, that you'll receive a more thorough, kinder treatment because you're paying for it. This has not been my experience. It *is* usually quicker to see someone or get a scan, but the *quality* of care is just as mixed as it is in the NHS, and paradoxically some of the more unpleasant encounters have been ones I've paid for. Private medicine does not necessarily mean better, more efficient or more caring, but it *does* mean a profit-based stance on everything.

So before you get your purse out, here is some advice from someone who has spent *a lot* on seeing people:

- **Research them**: look for qualifications, credentials, patient testimonies, experience.
- **Don't assume they will be better or different doctors just because you're paying**: they are often the same doctors you'll see in the NHS, you'll just see them a few months sooner.
- **You don't have unlimited time**: appointments might be slightly longer privately, but it's not guaranteed. I have often paid for half an hour but been hurried out in five minutes.
- **The answers might not be different**: it's very frustrating when it's cost you hundreds of pounds and you are told the same information.
- **Beware of hidden costs**: ask for a price estimate if they send you for additional tests/treatment. (Watch out for people 'upselling' tests/treatments, the ones you don't really need.)
- **You can always walk away from their advice/treatment**: one time I was so desperate I nearly agreed to pay £8,000 every six months for the rest of my life for a brainwave machine that would 'zap the pain responses'. This is *one* opinion, you don't have to buy it.
- **There are a lot of charlatans out there**: if they're selling you a 'fix' be very cautious. Every expert is clear; more research and analysis is required and there is currently no one solution. They might be able to alleviate some of the symptoms but no one has a cure at the moment.
- **Don't always believe them**: misdiagnosis can happen even when you've entered your credit card details. I've had doctors tell me that the disease and pain is due to fibromyalgia, bipolar, possible sexual trauma when I was younger, none of which are true.

- **They're not necessarily the 'best in the biz'**: they may be in a nice building with a posh postcode, but it doesn't mean that *they* are the best. It's not like in other jobs where you get the great office because you worked hard; you just need enough money to rent the room.

The endometriosis jigsaw

If the symptoms are persistent we can become completely absorbed in trying to resolve the problem, working on the assumption that, 'There must be a solution, I just haven't found it yet.' There is a great deal of contradictory information available, lots of scary stories and myths and it can be dizzying when even the experts say different things. We clutch at a piece of knowledge from here and a bit of advice from there; it's like trying to make a jigsaw without knowing what the picture is meant to be. It's not unusual to end up feeling drained and confused.

Western society works on the belief that we can get hold of everything, go anywhere, do anything. We have come to believe there is always a way to sort things: 'Because you're worth it'. If a dress doesn't fit you take it back; if there isn't a flight there must be another way of getting there. We live in a world were we can make the impossible possible. So it's not surprising that women with a difficult disease like endometriosis approach the condition in the same way. Except the quest is not for the right dress, it's for our health, our past selves and our future selves that need to feel better. If only we could find our guy, the right medication, the right surgery, the right combination of diet, pills and powders then it will all be OK. This is what leads to the decision to spend thousands of pounds on specialists and tests – even when you don't really have the money to do so. The quest goes on and on until *you* can't. It's expensive and disappointing and it's exhausting when you've exhausted all the options.

At least you have your health . . . (age 28–32)

My parents and I are going hog-wild throwing money at the problem. We're not rich, but any spare money goes on this, there has to be a way to get me better. I'm seeing specialists (for second, third, even fifth opinions), alternative therapists, psychologists, nutritionists, acupuncturists, herbalists, hypno-therapists, yoga teachers, pain specialists, even psychiatrists. I find myself in room after room begging for help. Many are cowboys offering quasi-cures or inaccurate diagnoses, taking advantage of people at their lowest and most vulnerable. But it doesn't stop me going to the next person. The problem is, when you're struggling this much you would do or take pretty much anything. This is the exact moment you need to be your best advocate, your most brilliant detective, but this is also the moment you cannot gather the strength to be that incisive.

Searching for a fix took over my life. I traipsed all over the country to see people. I was juggling work, trying to hide the effects of a mad hormone treatment and seeing five or six specialists a week. There is nothing I didn't try. I became my own guinea pig, my own science experiment. I wasted hours of my life trying to find 'the one' who would be able to sort me out. The Internet became a temptation I couldn't ignore and I'd google into the night, clicking on blue link after blue link. Going down these rabbit holes of hypochondria almost always made me feel worse.

I read books and websites and anything I could find.
I tried things suggested by friends and fellow sufferers on forums.
I drank special teas (they tasted rank).
I changed my diet again (bored!).
I tried to do more exercise (ouch).
I rattled around full of expensive vitamins.
I learnt about chakras and the 'colours' of my body.
I was belittled and disbelieved.
I was hypnotised and patronised and terrified.
I had sucky cups all over my back.
I dripped pipettes of CBD oil under my tongue.
I bobbed around in floatation tanks paid for by loving friends.
I took new painkillers and paid for trial drugs.
I had needles stuck everywhere (this helped).
I had MRI and CT scans, blood tests and ultrasounds.
I even let one guy 'talk' to my body, which didn't do much,
    but I felt a bit calmer after a lie-down.

Some things were very helpful, many were of no use to me
or their impact didn't last long enough to be worth the cost.
But engaging with the symptoms and trying to lessen them
did make me feel empowered and more hopeful and eventually I found a combination of things that helped.

How do you manage the symptoms then?

Most women with endometriosis are able to work around the symptoms, almost unconsciously sometimes, and it's a successful strategy
for much of the time. I was one of these women for many years,
but there were also bad days when I found it hard to deal with the

symptoms, especially those caused by medications, so I looked into other ways to manage them. Over the years I have tried many things that have provided much relief and often made it possible to live without (even) more medication. In my experience, it's never just one thing but a combination of things that gets you out of a pickle, and this applies to long-term illness too. In terms of managing pain, this is what pelvic-pain specialist Katy Vincent told me:

> People tend to get better if we do lots of things at the same time, rather than trying this and then that; it's a bit of a perfect storm. Your muscles are in spasm, your nerves are irritated. Every time you have a period your muscles are more in spasm and your nerves become more irritated. So every month that flares it up, every time you have sex that flares it up, your nerves are irritated, that flares it up. If we don't damp down all of those bits there is usually enough to maintain that cycle, so we have to try three or four things at once.

THINGS I KNOW NOW

- There is no one-size-fits-all model to manage endometriosis; you might have to try a few things to find what works for you. Recommendations are useful if you're not sure where to begin.

- Think about what you can do to increase your strength, energy and better health (you're not going to like this but it includes diet and some gentle exercise).

- Do you need more emotional/psychological support? Psychotherapy, counselling, hypnotherapy, mindfulness?

- Have you considered any alternative/holistic therapies that might help?

- If symptoms or pain are worse at particular points in your cycle, think about what strategies would be most useful at those times. A PMS massage or a pain-relieving acupuncture session?

Alternative medicine

I'm a big fan of alternative medicine as my friends who have been advised to 'Pop some arnica on that' or 'Smear some yogurt on this' will tell you. But I know others may be more sceptical. The dismissal of alternative therapies is mainly because there isn't much to support their efficacy scientifically yet, but this doesn't mean they might not work for you. Acupuncture, for example, has had mixed efficacy in medical trials but is something which helps many women manage the symptoms and pain that can come with endometriosis. Others find massage or reflexology helpful. Some believe that complementary medicine is a placebo, that the effects are psychological: our desire for it to work is why it works, but if you feel the benefits from a treatment, who cares?

Here are some things that lots of women use to alleviate symptoms:

Acupuncture	Homeopathy	NLP (neuro-linguistic
Reflexology	Osteopathy	programming)
Herbal medicine	Hypnotherapy	Autogenic training
Chinese medicine	Massage	

THINGS I KNOW NOW

- You may need patience to find out what's useful for you and it can be frustrating to spend money on things that don't work.

- Ask friends if for recommendations, and research the qualifications and reviews for alternative practitioners.

- Anything that reduces stress and aids relaxation, even for a few hours, is worth doing. It helps to regulate your body and mind, which will make it easier for you to handle pain and other symptoms caused by the disease or treatments.

- Alternative medicine looks at you as a whole, which helps with the various effects endometriosis can have on the rest of your body.

- It's worth asking your doctor (and the alternative therapist) whether some complementary therapies may interact with the more traditional medical treatments you might be taking.

- Appointments are usually a bit longer – around an hour so there is time for the practitioner to listen; feeling that you're being heard is important, especially if you're suffering a myriad of things without much support – sympathy and validation alone often provides some relief.

- It can be very tiring trying to manage symptoms *and* your life. A little time out to rest and recoup revitalises hope, enables you to recharge much faster and keep going.

For me, acupuncture, cranial massage and reflexology have provided the most relief when I've been on hormonal treatments. Deep-tissue massage helps to relax my system, which gives me respite so I can harness my strength. NLP hypnotherapy and mindfulness meditation help reduce anxiety and the physical tension in the rest of my body caused by pain.

Lifestyle changes

There are lots of thing *you* can do to manage the symptoms in conjunction with, or for some women instead of, taking medications. I know first hand how overwhelming it can feel when someone suggests overhauling your life for this condition; you might not want to, you might not have the energy to make these changes right now, or you might be trying to ignore it all, hoping it goes away. However, I know now that engaging with the symptoms can give you a sense of control and empowerment. There is nothing stronger than actively doing something to make yourself feel better. This part of the book looks at what you might be able to do to alleviate some of the effects of endometriosis if they are having an effect on your day-to-day life.

These Things Will Exacerbate the Symptoms

- **Not enough sleep and eating badly.**
- **High levels of adrenaline**: annoyingly this can come after lots of fun too.
- **Stress**: at work, disputes with friends, relationship problems and break-ups, bereavement, illness.
- **Mental-health issues**: anxiety, excessive worrying, depression.
- **Excessive physical activity**: exercise can be helpful but it might be about balance, try not to overdo it. TIP: this is especially important post-op, it takes time to get full strength back.
- **Sitting in one position for a long time**: e.g. flights, trains, driving, theatre, cinema; try to move around in the chair if you can't get up.
- **Lots of travelling/long journeys**: can make you very tired, try to allow for this if possible, e.g. set aside a day for rest on arrival?
- **Not enough hydration**: especially if you're taking lots of painkillers or are somewhere hot. The extra stress on your system can make you dizzy or nauseous.

> • **Wheat, gluten and alcohol**: they're inflammatory so can put added pressure on your system. TIP: If you *do* have alcohol, avoid very acidic or wheat-based drinks.
>
> What a cheerful list! I only mention it because I'm about to tell you what might help . . .

Now I have to stop eating everything I like too?

You've got a condition that causes pain and sometimes incapacitates you? What do you do next? That's right, you cut out everything you enjoy as well: alcohol, caffeine, sugar, stodgy comfort food, dairy. We know that these things can aggravate the symptoms, so it's best to avoid or minimise them, but it's hard not to feel like you're depriving yourself. When people suggested I overhaul my diet followed by 'Why wouldn't you do something that might make you feel better?' I resisted it. I didn't want to close off *every* avenue of fun. To tell someone that they ought to do things that will make their life even *less* pleasurable when they're already having a difficult time is infuriating. I knew that what I ate would have consequences, but I wasn't ready to give up any more for this disease. After operation three, Dr B advised I look at alternative ways to manage the symptoms in addition to the medical things he could offer. He suggested a book called *Endometriosis: a Key to Healing and Fertility Through Nutrition* by Dian Shepperson Mills, an endometriosis and nutrition expert. The idea is to follow an anti-inflammatory diet to reduce your symptoms, and in particular pain. Once I had read about how this diet could alleviate some of the symptoms, I couldn't ignore it. Now I could hear this critical voice in my head saying, 'You're not helping yourself shovelling biscuits and pizzas and buckets of Kentucky, are you? No wonder you feel ill!' Like any lifestyle change, you have to be ready to commit to it, and be motivated to continue – now it had got to the point where I would try anything to feel better.

Tupperware and Room service (age 19)

I've been wandering around the supermarket for an hour with my dad trying to work out what the hell I can eat. One of the major changes is that I don't have wheat or gluten anymore and I'm getting increasingly depressed and agitated – it's in *everything*. I'm hungry all the time, like biting my own hand, black spots in my eyes, frantic hungry. I've only been doing it for two weeks and I can't get full up. Why haven't the doctors been able to fix it? What was the point of all the surgeries and drugs if they're not working?

* * *

Two months later

I've been doing the diet for two months but I am still struggling to work out what I can have and how to make it work when so much of my life is spontaneous and without routine. I'm staying at a hotel with my mum and I've just ordered room service for the first time in my life, some gnocchi is on its way and I'm salivating as I wait. This shaky feeling where you can't think about anything but food is what my family describes as 'the bonk'. It can be used as follows: 'Sorry I'm stuffing my face with all this ham from the fridge, I've got the bonk.' The food arrives and I wolf it down. Within the hour I'm in a foetal position on the bed, with a pounding head-ache, writhing around like I have food poisoning. It turns out gnocchi has a coating of flour so that probably explains it. Who knew you could become intolerant so quickly?

* * *

Four years later

I'm at my cousin's wedding. I've been gluten-free for a while now, so I know what's coming: a *really* tasteless chicken option without sauce or flavour, just to be sure I won't sue them if I go into anaphylactic shock. I won't of course, I'm not coeliac, but most people don't know the difference between allergic and intolerant so they cover their backs. It's hard to explain to people that you have caused your own intolerance by cutting something from your diet; that you have actively made life a bit harder for yourself and anyone catering for you. But I feel so much better not eating it. I'm lighter, less bloated and lethargic and because I'm more conscious of what I'm eating, my diet is better than ever. I don't grab food without thinking any more which means I have lost weight too – bonus!

While waiting for the food to be served, a woman at our table starts to take out various-sized Tupperware boxes from her bag. As the boxes mount up it becomes clear she has brought nearly an entire meal's worth of food with her, including her own gravy granules. We listen in amazement as she delivers a monologue about the variety of intolerances she's burdened with: 'Anything with eggs, anything that's pasteurised, anything that isn't pasteurised enough, dairy . . .' On and on she went. This level of fuss around food irks me and I resolve to never be like this, to never talk about it as if it were an extension of my personality. When I go to a wedding or out for dinner I will quietly mention my dietary requirements but if there isn't an alternative I'll just eat what I can. It gives me a sense of control. I can change my diet but not let it change who I am.

Wheat-free wisdom

I've been wheat-free for fourteen years now and it has been the most effective management for my symptoms (other than surgery). And although I have never stopped missing pizza, croissants and naan bread, I would highly recommend it. It's hard to cut things out completely and it can be expensive to get alternatives or substitutes for things, but it's worth exploring this particular lifestyle change to help manage your symptoms.

Within six months of being very strict about the diet I felt such a change. I realised I'd got used to feeling blown up like I was full of air or, on the worst days, rocks. Being less heavy and swollen also made moving around and exercise easier and I wasn't as tired either. After a process of trial and error I became more relaxed about it, allowing a few things back in like coffee, the occasional splash of soy sauce, some dairy, but sticking to the principles of an anti-inflammatory diet.

- No wheat or gluten
- Reduced meat, particularly red meat
- No packaged sauces or ready meals
- Reduce as much sugar and salt in diet as possible
- Oily fish three times a week (omega 3 and 6 are good)

- No or reduced dairy
- Fresh food when possible
- No coffee or tea – caffeine aggravates the pain (reduce if you can't cut)
- No or reduced alcohol

In essence the idea is to have a balanced, nutritious diet. You can have some treats but everything should be in moderation and if you recognise certain foods make you feel worse, avoid them. Dian's book is a great introduction to the concepts of the diet, it has meal suggestions and inspiring stories from other women with endometriosis who have benefitted from the nutrition route. It might feel too daunting a task to undertake when you're feeling poorly and tired, or it might feel as if removing certain foods would take away some of your much-needed joy. If this is the case, just be aware of it and perhaps reduce your intake of 'inflammatory' foods a little when you can, as it could really help you.

I might try it – what do I need to know?
- It requires a bit of attention when you're planning meals initially but once you're in the mindset, it becomes much easier to do. You see very quickly what you can have on a menu or in a shop and you ignore what you can't.
- There are many more substitutes available than you think, but some stuff is nicer than others, so you might need to try things until you find what you like.
- Experiment with making your own stuff if you can as many of the shop-bought alternatives contain high levels of sugar. It also keeps costs down if you can cook your own versions of things as substitutes can be expensive.
- What is the difference between wheat-free and gluten-free?

This doesn't matter if you're not allergic, but for the purposes of cutting it out for inflammatory reasons, it's best to avoid both. (TIP: It's easier to say 'gluten-free' in restaurants; learn how to say it in other languages for when you travel.)

• One little joy is that you can warrant lashings of butter/sauce/toppings on the 'bread' because it's so dry.

Vitamins and immune-system support

Vitamins don't resolve the endometriosis itself, but they help to support your system and provide a good base to fight off other ailments. The disease can have an impact on your immune system so it's good to have a high vitamin content in addition to a good diet. Always speak to a qualified nutritionist for guidance on what vitamins you might need and tell your doctor that you're taking supplements too so as to be sure nothing is interacting with any medications.

THINGS I KNOW NOW

If you're going to get vitamins buy the best quality you can afford. You need high strength and no added yeast, wheat, etc. They might be expensive but you need them to be this good for them to work. Your body is already fighting a disease and inflammation so you need them to be strong to support your whole system.

Exercise and endometriosis

When I read things about how women with endometriosis should exercise, that we should muster up our inner strength and try to go for a run or do a gym session, I want to throw my phone at the wall. *You* try even bending to tie the laces of your trainers when you're in this much pain. Muster yourself! It's not uncommon to feel isolated, jealous and guilty when we see other sufferers talking of marathons and strength, especially if your brain wants to do it but your body simply can't. But over time I recognised that on the days when you're feeling stronger, the right (gentle) exercise can be very helpful for managing not only the physical symptoms but also your mental and emotional well-being. You might have to monitor how much physical activity you do in order to conserve energy and not aggravate the pain. There may be certain times where it feels impossible to do much physically at all but it's important not to stop moving all together and allow pain in one area or the symptoms of this condition to stop you using the rest of your body.

THINGS I KNOW NOW

- The key is not to overdo it; build up your activity.

- Try to be proud of what you have achieved (even if it seems less than you used to do). Choose something you actually *like*; it makes it easier to motivate yourself.

- Find something that works for *you*: gentle yoga, walking, swimming, the gym even. This is about what's right for *your* body not what anyone else is telling you.

- Moving around and exercise helps to brush away some of the 'endometriosis fog' and cloudy fatigue from painkillers.

Bench (age 15-32)

I was always told to be as active as I would normally be when I was on my period, but most of the time this was impossible. Mine didn't feel like normal cramps that would be eased by a few lengths or some stretching. I felt so ill I thought I'd be sick or faint if I moved at all. I just needed to curl up; still and warm like a cat. On the bad days at school when we had PE, I sat on benches with my knees clenched to my chest. I never had letters to excuse me but the teachers couldn't ignore my pale, green face and my fragile body leaning and squirming in pain.

As time went on and my friends started their periods, I couldn't understand how they could play tennis or run when I could barely stand up. I felt embarrassed that I wasn't strong enough to drag myself up to join them.

When I got older, I just avoided doing anything *really* active if I was bleeding. And when the pain became constant (not just cyclical) I tried to avoid anything physical that wasn't totally necessary because I thought extra exertion would make it worse. I'd gone from many years of too much activity and not enough rest, to the complete opposite. I would wake up and everything hurt, like I was bruised or had run for hours the previous day. I'd have to ease myself out of bed by rolling to one side and wait patiently for an hour until the painkillers kicked in and my body stopped pounding. I was in my early thirties; this had to stop. With the help of various pelvic-pain physiotherapists and yoga teachers, I started to do very gentle exercise again. I began with tiny movements that were tailored to the scar tissue and nerve damage in my abdomen, building up (the right kind of) strength in my pelvis and loosening the muscles that had, over the years, knotted around to protect me, like the thorns in *Sleeping Beauty*. The muscle and nerve memories were ingrained so took time to reverse. I'd been adapting my posture to ease and work around the pain; sitting and standing badly, overusing my upper-back muscles, curling my shoulders in a hunch and holding myself awkwardly. Progress was slow, but over time it got easier, I built strength and released tension. I also learnt stretches that can be used on the worst days and ones to calm my body when it's in panic mode because I've done too much.

THINGS I KNOW NOW

- Gentle stretching and exercise are really important when you have persistent pain as everything becomes wound up, tight and tense.

- The earlier you get into good pelvic habits the better.

- Regulating your breathing and using your body is really important, ignoring pain or muscular issues connected to pain is not a great idea. There are things you can do to alleviate these issues so you don't increase the ailments and amount of things your body is dealing with.

- Yoga – child's pose in a bath on the bad days is great for lower-back pain. Cat-Cow poses are also very useful and help with anxiety too.

I can't get no sleep

Pain, anxiety and medication can all affect sleep and if you don't get enough, or enough of the deep stuff, there can be a knock-on effect to your immune system, mental health, mood and pain. It's not uncommon to find it hard to get to sleep but then impossible to wake up in the morning, especially if the night-time medications make you groggy. Painkillers can also send you into a strange combination of tired and wired. If you mismanage them, you can find yourself wide awake at 2.30 a.m., engrossed in a Bette Midler documentary and wondering why you're not in bed like everyone else.

If your sleep is being affected, there are some things that can help:

- **Look at your bedtime routine and make some adaptions**: could you go to bed earlier? Wake up earlier? Is the room too bright? Are you looking at screens before bed?
- **Plan your intake of painkillers**: rather than just taking them as and when. This gives you more control over 'spikes' and reduces frustration if pain is interrupting your sleep.
- **Tinker with your drugs**: if pain is keeping you awake. Try taking painkillers at different times, so you can sleep through. Getting the balance of enough sleep but also being able to wake up in the morning may take a little time.
- **Speak to your doctor**: if sleep becomes a persistent problem.

If you're suffering from insomnia due to various medications or anxiety, it can develop into a pattern of sleeping in later and later. Realistically this is not an option for most people because we have to go to work, so we begin to live on very little sleep and feel increasingly lousy.

- **Re-regulate your sleep**: break the cycle by changing your routine in increments. Rather than trying to get up very early to jump-start your system, wake up ten minutes earlier tomorrow, and then the next day, and so on, until you're back to your regular sleep regime.

One pain specialist told me that our brains really love routines and patterns, so the more you repeat them, the better you'll feel. However, it can be hard to stick to a routine if you have a busy life, or travel for work, etc. So here are some things that might help and some can be used wherever you lay your head:

- **Maternity pillow/pillow between your legs**: reduces strain on abdominal muscles and lower back, curl into it.
- **Hypnotherapy/meditation on your phone**: use wireless head-phones/a wireless headband with speakers so you can drift to sleep without getting tangled in the wires.
- **Clean sheets, good bedding and pyjamas**: comfort and hygiene are really important.
- **Electric blanket**: warmth is great, especially if you're tense or have lower-back pain.
- **Calming fragrances**: lavender, bergamot – sprayed on pillows or in a diffuser.

Just relax! Easy to say, right, but here are some things that will help calm your system before sleeping:

- **Focus on your breathing:** in for three beats, out for three.
- **Scan your body, feet to face:** concentrate on relaxing the muscles and let go of the tension (especially in neck, jaw and face, they can become tight if you're in pain a lot).

- **Focus on the good stuff:** think of some positive rather than negative things that have happened during the day. If thinking about your day is stressful then switch to something you're looking forward to instead.

Mindfulness

Being told to be 'mindful' or 'in the present' can be exasperating if your present is something you want to escape. Being 'in the moment' when you're in pain feels like the worst place to be, *but* it works. Here's why:

- Think about a delicious chocolate ice cream? Really imagine it. The taste? The texture? Is it in a tub or a cone?
- Now think about anything else but you're not allowed to think about that ice cream. It's hard to take you mind off it, isn't it?

Similarly with pain, even with distraction or determination you can't *completely* ignore it. Your brain is using up a lot of energy trying to ignore it (mind-over-matter) and it puts a lot of pressure on your central nervous system. Your body is in 'alert' or 'fight' mode and therefore you have a heightened sensitivity and respond to everything in an urgent way as though it's a threat. This then adds to the stress, anxiety, exhaustion and, ironically, the pain. Distractions can be a very useful strategy when you have persistent pain, but if the signals are very strong it can be hard to ignore them (see Chapter 13 to understand why).

The Present (age 29)

Everyone is telling me 'Live in the present', but I can't. My head swings from future to past but will not stand still in the here and now because it is intolerable. I just need this pain to stop. The only present I *want* is something nice to cheer me up. The meditation apps I've tried seem to be making it even worse; it's a heightened sensory experience where I can't even escape my head. A friend suggests NLP hypnosis and I meet a kind woman who listens, is gentle and tailors the hypnosis to me. She gives me CDs of the sessions. I download them to my phone and use them on long journeys, in bed, at lunchtime, if my boss shouts too much. It helps. I sleep better and it's reducing the tension and anxiety that come with the pain, but I don't think this is the 'present' everyone's talking about . . .

* * *

One of my doctors declares that Western medicine might have hit a wall now for me and he suggests I try acupuncture, herbal medicine or this magic chair he's heard about recently. It does something with sound waves and aids meditation apparently. It's not that I am sceptical about the mind–body connection or the idea that mood affects the pain levels, but I just can't get the mindfulness thing to work for me. I decide to try it anyway, why not. After several sessions in the Zen Satori chair (a vibroacoustic technology that assists deep relaxation) I begin to feel the benefits of focused breathing and meditation. I feel lighter and restored, but the sessions are expensive. I download the audio tracks as a guide so I can do it at home, but without the vibrations. I start to do it every day and it feels more cumulative in its effects than other therapies, my body feels calmer and my mental health has improved. I like the fact I have this new thing I can do, that it's ready to go on the bad days, it gives me a sense of control – like another tool in my pain management toolbox. Within a few months meditation becomes a vital coping strategy during flare-ups or stress. It might not stop the pain but it helps to calm everything down so the pain doesn't 'spike' so much during stressful times.

I asked Stefan Chmelik, acupuncturist, herbal physician and mindfulness guru, why I found meditation so hard initially.

Mindfulness is 'awareness of the self in the present moment without judgement'. We could say that stress and anxiety are awareness of self in the present moment but *with* judgement. For someone who is afraid of how their body feels, being asked to feel and experience their internal world can be very frightening.

That might explain why I struggled with it so much at first. I had another question for Stefan: why is meditation particularly useful for someone with long-term pain or illness?

Excess adrenaline and other stress hormones in the body are short-acting pro-inflammatory chemicals produced to create super-reactive states. When in emergency flight-fight-freeze mode, the body is not in a position to do much more than react. It is well established that deep breathing and meditation lead to increased stress resilience and better balance of stress hormone activity.

So that's that. Get crossing those legs and breathing in (and out).

12

Body matters

When you have been living with a body that causes pain or physically changes because of the treatments, your relationship with it can be altered significantly. The hormonal interventions can also have a huge impact on your mood, and mental health. It's hard not to become enemies with a body that is inconsistent and unpredictable. You can stop trusting or relying on it and become fearful of what it might do next. If nothing else, just planning your life around the symptoms can be enough to make you feel frustrated and irritable.

Living with endometriosis can also affect self-confidence and over time it may lead to a development of a dysfunctional, distanced relationship with your body, perhaps even a critical internal monologue that is impatient and angry. If you are missing out on important work or social activities, or you lose relationships indirectly or directly due to health problems, this can also increase resentment towards your body.

Detached (age 31)

I am aware that detachment from my body has been developing over time. It's like there are two versions of me: the one that's busy, bright and stays up late; and the other who needs constant reassurance that I'm listening, that I'm paying attention and if I don't give it enough, it will make sure I remember to by spiking the pain. I buy something lovely to cheer up the first one whose life is being disrupted by the second. But treats stop being treats if you do them all the time. I have started to view endometriosis as a punishing force coming in to spoil everything and I'm not going to let it. So I shut off my body and focus on my mind, it's a nicer place to be. I think of my body like a derelict stately home when you can't afford the repairs, so you board up some of the rooms and forget about them, living in the few rooms kept open while the rest slowly decays around you. But the mind and body need to be in sync, you can't put the body on the naughty step and hope it shuts up, it won't. You've got to open the rooms up and be in the whole house, even if you don't like some of the rooms.

THINGS I KNOW NOW

- Although you may have become suspicious and untrusting of your body, you have to keep reminding yourself that this is *one* issue. Your body isn't broken or weak, in fact I'll tell you now, you're actually *very strong.*

- Don't ignore other ailments or issues that may arise along-side endometriosis, you don't have to feel unwell all the time, ask for more help.

- Invest in your body: good diet, vitamins, sleep, comfort, anything that makes you feel better, even temporarily, is worth trying.

It would be funny if I weren't so embarrassed . . .

'They sent me to the women's clinic. I never knew there were so many ways for women to fall to pieces. They've got their bosoms hanging out, pelvic floors dangling, there's a woman with her cervix in a margarine tub, and she's saying 'I took it out to wash it but I couldn't get it back in!'

Victoria Wood, *At It Again* (2001)

You can't help but lose any inhibitions you might have had once you've had endometriosis for some time. Within a couple of minutes you're telling a complete stranger the most intimate details about your sex life and toilet habits (it's usually a doctor, not just someone at a bus stop). There are suddenly a lot of questions about your body that you don't want to *think* about, let alone say out loud. You have to talk candidly about how often you go for a wee, how much you bleed, whether you vomit; no bodily function is too personal to discuss. I'm not particularly embarrassed by this stuff, but even *I* feel uncomfortable talking about it. Unfortunately, part of the process of getting the right support is that you *have* to discuss these things and after a while being embarrassed stops being such a concern as there are more important things at stake. It gets to a point when you've been through some of the most humiliating moments you could imagine and survived. I'm now even able to laugh about them. Here are some of my favourites:

- Weeing in a plastic cup, then sitting in the waiting room trying to hide it up your sleeve without tipping it all over yourself.
- When doctors ask loudly: 'And when did you last have penetrative sex?' (Will someone please tell them that the curtains are *not* soundproof!)
- People knocking on doors and then coming in regardless of the response, while your legs are spread-eagled in stirrups mid-scan.
- Your most private parts being discussed in corridors, in front of porters and other patients; while you're still putting your knickers back on.

There's always time for a laugh

Proof that this is true, is when a young, attractive, male doctor asks if he can do a rectal exam, 'Is it OK if I stick my finger up your back passage?' and I have to fight the urge to say, 'Well usually someone buys me a drink first!'

Laughing at something helps to reduce some of the tension in the moment, provides perspective and gives you back a bit of control.

If I have learnt one thing over the last twenty years it's that finding a laugh, even in the darkest times, is the best way to

---

cope and distract yourself during long scans, uncomfortable tests and flare-ups. Going to a happier place makes it all a bit easier; mine involves funny things or a better way to tell a joke. For instance, using the example above; I try to think of other punchlines in response to the doctor's question:

'Should we ask my husband to step out of the room?'
'Is this something I could do at home?'
'Will you be using a glove?'
And the classic – 'Well, that's all very well, Doctor, but it's my ear that's the problem.'

There are still many secrets when it comes to what it's *really* like to live with endometriosis, which is understandable as it can be deeply disconcerting and shocking to acknowledge some of the effects the disease and treatments can have on you. Sometimes *not* talking about it is a coping mechanism, perhaps hoping that by not saying it out loud it will go away or not be true. But after *too long,* I started to ask for help and I realised suffering in silence wasn't necessary because there are things that can be done to alleviate some of this stuff.

She's talking shit again!

Discussing the details of your bowel movements is excruciatingly embarrassing. Even after all these years I still find it the most awkward part to talk about, because no one talks about it! It would have really helped me to have known about this stuff, that I wasn't the only one experiencing these things, so I'm going to talk about it now – hold tight!

Bowel pain may be caused by disease, but it could simply be that the inflammation in your pelvis makes it uncomfortable to open them. Constipation can also be a side effect of the medications or painkillers, and this, in turn, can make the pain worse. Ironic isn't it? But I don't remember Alanis Morissette singing about *this*, do you?

Over the years I have become much more familiar with phrases such as 'bunged up', 'a lot of congestion' and 'trapped wind' than I'd like. Doctors ask 'Is it soft, hard, large, extra large?' Like a meal at a fast-food restaurant? Or 'Is it very loose or little pellets of differing size?' Like a bag of Revels?

THINGS I KNOW NOW

Don't stay quiet about these symptoms. Your doctor will have seen and heard it all; they won't be squeamish or embarrassed. Bowel issues and rectal pain can be a really important symptoms that can help doctors assess if there is disease in certain places. They also have things that can ease this particular issue; you don't have to manage this on your own.

Dagger

No one knows the feeling of a dagger stabbing down through your ass like a woman with endometriosis. Man, that is like black-out, vomit-inducing painful isn't it? Urgent cramping, as though you've got serious food poisoning, all this pressure but then nothing is coming? I could have written a selection of short stories in the time I have spent rocking on a toilet, humming to calm my body and trying to focus during these bouts. Your vision goes blurry, your body gets very hot and you feel light-headed as though you're going to faint. I know, I'm strong, 'I am woman' and all that, but this is like trying to pass a boulder!

Constipation is one thing, but when it's diarrhoea *as well* as bleeding profusely and vomiting it feels like punishment indeed. All my orifices have turned against me; it's like having triplets and not enough hands. These are the times I wish I had something to knock me out completely. These are the parts of living with endometriosis that nobody sees.

THINGS I KNOW NOW

- **Lean forward**: so your hands and elbows are on your knees. It takes pressure off your bowel, rectum and bladder and reduces the strain on your abdominal muscles. This can help with urinary pain too.

- **Breathe into it**: I talk to myself, 'It's OK, you're OK, you know what this is.' It might sound (and feel) ridiculous but it helps calm my body and brain.

- **Try not to strain or push**: it can cause haemorrhoids or anal tags – then you'll have another thing to deal with!

Lax about laxatives

Trapped wind or constipation can really exacerbate the pain but part of making it better might mean your bowels are unreliable for a bit, which can be uncomfortable and embarrassing, so often we ignore it and hope it will go away on its own. It's also hard to know quite how fast the laxative process will be and worrying whether you'll make it to the toilet in time can be difficult to handle. There are natural ways to manage constipation: increasing fibre in your diet, taking psyllium husk, keeping hydrated. There are also the pharmaceutical things like Fybogel and Senokot that might help.

Prior to surgery you may be offered an enema; not having an impacted bowel makes it easier for them to operate. I don't know if you're familiar with them, but it's a bit like a fire drill in your colon, it's very much a case of 'everyone out'. It's a fast and furious treatment but it works well. Alternatively, your doctor may suggest a 'bowel prep' at home the day before surgery. This also works pretty fast, but you just keep going throughout the day and usually you aren't allowed to eat. I recommend you don't leave the house when you're taking this. Your bottom can get sore, you might feel a little light-headed, hungry and empty by bedtime. The good news is you can drink plenty of fluids and emptying your bowels completely may ease the pain a bit because your bowel won't be pressing on any inflammation in your pelvis.

> **THINGS I KNOW NOW**
>
> - A stool softener helps loosen without being urgent. Something like Lactulose is good; you can get it from a pharmacy without prescription.
>
> - Get some calendula cream or Vaseline for your bottom; it helps with soreness.
>
> - You may not be given an enema or bowel prep before surgery, but if possible try to avoid constipation before surgery as post-surgery it can be harder to push with the swelling.

And what about having sex? Well I'm a bit busy, Doctor, but if you think we have time?

I used to be baffled when doctors asked me if I had pain during sex. I never had, maybe a little after sometimes. This is another confusing thing about endometriosis: some women experience pain during or after intercourse, others don't, and some only experience discomfort at particular times in their cycle. Many women don't experience pain associated with sex itself but might have pain, inflammation or a susceptibility to UTIs after the event.

Over time this condition can also have an impact on how you feel about your body and your perceptions around desirability and self-esteem, which can put you off intimacy and sex. It's not surprising if the parts that are supposed to be pleasurable are causing you discomfort, pain and even embarrassment. It might be none of this; perhaps it's just that sometimes the pain is so great you stop feeling interested in sex altogether or that the hormonal treatments are affecting your libido. It's not uncommon to become so apprehensive about disrupting this unpredictable area of your body in case it increases the pain or other symptoms so you'd rather not do it.

Endometriosis might feel like it's spoiling *all* your fun if it's also affecting your sex life, but here are some things that might help.

Mission(ary) statements
- Explore positions; some might be less uncomfortable at particular times. Being in control of the depth and angle of penetration can help.
- What other sexual activities could you do if penetrative sex is not possible?
- TIP: it's less awkward if you talk about this with your partner before it gets to the hot and heavy bit.

Lube is queen
- It's not only fun (and heightens the pleasure for both of you), but it really helps if you have tension or less natural lubrication than usual (possible side effect of some medications).
- This is not a concession; loads of couples use lube, it's not because you're not excited, it's just a facilitator.
- TIP: try to get natural/organic lubes rather than scented ones as they can aggravate an already sensitive area, disrupt your delicate PH balance and cause inflammation.

It's not you (or them)

- **Libido can be affected by**: hormones, endometriosis, medication and your mental and emotional well-being.
- **Try to find a way to talk about it**: what might you be able to do together? What might make you more comfortable? Communication really helps reduce confusion and anxiety around this stuff.
- **Don't lose out on *all* intimacy**: cuddle, massage, hand stuff. It doesn't always have to be about orgasms (though I know they're great).
- **Speak to your doctor**: about changing medications (particularly birth control) if this is having a significant impact on sex drive.

Impossible

If you've been suffering with pain and had surgical and hormonal interventions for some time, it is no wonder things feel tight and inflamed. The muscles in the pelvic region can become tense because your body has been responding to a 'threat' for so long. The good news is, it doesn't have to stay this way and with time and the right help you can find something that works for you. I spoke to Katy Vincent, a pain specialist at the Endometriosis CaRe Centre, Oxford University, about how you can reduce and reverse pain signals in this area:

> Pain with sex is not uncommon. The nervous system has memories and nerves can change their behaviour so they can fire at a lower threshold. We get better results with physiotherapy if we use a nerve painkiller at the same time, which damps down how sensitive the nervous system is because otherwise you touch the skin and muscles go into spasm in response. If you can get that area not to be so sensitive then we can start working on the muscles.

For some women the pain that comes during or after sex is too much, even the *thought* of having sex worsens the pain. If you're abstaining but desperately want this bit of your life back, try to see a pelvic-pain physiotherapist, and perhaps even look into psychosexual counselling support too. There are also items that can help you to get back to the right kind of sensitivity (there's a link to a great company called Pelvic Relief on page 342).

Marilyn Monroe and Me

Did you know that Marilyn Monroe had endometriosis? When I read about this in my early twenties it changed everything. Reading about the effect it had on her life made me very sad; she had pain so bad she became reliant on barbiturates and she experienced grief around fertility (she had several miscarriages and an ectopic pregnancy). But I also found a strange solace knowing she had what I had, because not only had she been successful and brilliant, she was also one of the sexiest women to have ever lived. Knowing this really helped me to separate the disease and my sexuality.

Image and confidence

I don't hate my body. There are many bits I rather like. I just wish it were a bit more reliable and fun to be with. I have been over-conscious about how my body looks from a young age, perhaps in retrospect right back from the age of nine. Becoming a woman happened overnight; I went to bed a little girl and woke up an adolescent. I don't think that's possible but it did feel quick. I was awkward and a bit chubby, not quite tall enough yet for my new wide hips, big bottom and breasts. I didn't feel carefree and light any more, I was a child in an increasingly adult body. Scratches of purple and white ran up my thighs and bottom, mostly fading over time to fine, silvery, sandworm lines. But my inner thighs still look like tigers have been at them; beauticians stare, worried that these are the scars of a self-harmer. Smoking, prescription drugs and falling in love with assholes is the only self-harming I ever did. These? These are a result of growing up too fast. What I didn't realise at the time was that, for me, some of these bodily changes also came with a disease.

She's let herself go a bit these days hasn't she? (age 30)

The only positive thing about endometriosis for me was that it wasn't visible. No one needed to know unless I wanted to tell them. As an actor it meant I could play characters that didn't have this dark storm going on inside, as a person I got some control because I didn't *have* to talk about it. I got really good at hiding the symptoms too. I learnt what I could manage: what heels were too high to function, what painkillers reacted with alcohol, the precision timing of taking them and how many drinks I could have. I learnt how to differentiate between nausea and when I was actually going to be sick, so I could get to the toilet quickly enough. I learnt to carry tampons, pads and painkillers in *every* bag, always. It was a vital part of my mental health that I looked well, that I appeared to be normal, so people didn't ask about it all the time and I didn't have to *be* the disease.

When the pain meant I was unable to work as a comedian, I became quite depressed. Visually I appeared fine, a bit more make-up, no more heels. The only things giving me away were that I was leaning on stuff or sitting down a bit more. I stopped eating much; I wasn't hungry but I also felt nauseous and food seemed to make the pain worse. I became very thin, a combination of stress, heartbreak and virtually no appetite. 'You look great – so thin! How do you do it?' 'A diet of codeine, coffee and cigarettes!' But I was only half-joking. 'But you're not ill-thin are you?' I think they meant life-threatening ill. I felt ridiculous saying, 'Well, I have this thing with my uterus . . .'

I quite liked being so thin. The pain was easier because I wasn't carting loads of weight around and I could wear really tight clothes without worrying about rolls when I sat down or lumps under my bra. My body *hurt* but for the first time ever I liked how it *looked*. Extreme weight loss is noticed by people, but there aren't many compliments when it goes the other way. Things were about to change radically.

* * *

I can't hide endometriosis any more; suddenly I *look* ill. These hefty hormones are affecting everything: my weight is increasing rapidly, my hair is falling out, my nails split and my skin is dry and scaly. My eyes have lost their sparkle; they are just big, heavy, dark blobs around tired sockets. I go wild in shops, spending money I haven't got in an attempt to find comfort in clothes and anything that might make me feel normal and halfway attractive.

We have a penchant for 'chub' in our family, we go to plump easily and quickly given the chance. But this isn't like normal weight gain; this is 'pudge'. That's right, I've made up a word. A combination of podgy and chub, that is the only way to describe this swollen, shiny, stretched skin. Regardless of how much matte make-up I pile on, I still look like an over-filled, raw sausage.

My swollen fingers are too big for my rings, my puffy face accentuates my pointy chin and my legs look like the large hams that hang in the windows of Italian delicatessens. On holiday they rub together in the heat. I get sore patches and we have to buy dressings and tape them to my thighs. My mother, thirty-four years older than I am, runs and climbs and plays with her grandchildren. I lean on a rock. I feel ancient, like my body is shutting down bit by bit.

I look in the mirror; who is this person all flabby, pale and bloated, so round, so *ill*? 'But how do you feel in yourself?' I don't. I don't feel like myself. This isn't my body any more. My confidence is on the floor. I've got a wedding to go to but I feel so horrible and I *look* so horrible that, for the first time in my life, I'm considering not going to something because I have nothing to wear. My friend Rose takes me shopping for a dress, she's calm and puts lots of breaks in to sit down and laugh. Eventually we find something I feel sort of comfortable in. Rose is a dream friend for many reasons, but this was one of the kindest practical things someone could have done for me when I was so ill, and something I didn't have the strength to do on my own.

* * *

I'm getting bigger and bigger and I'm so uncomfortable that it's getting to the point where I just want to live in dungarees. Exercise is too painful so all I can do is reduce what I eat, but I'm already down to corn cakes, salads and 'light' everything. I wouldn't mind if I was eating tubs of chocolate of an evening but I'm sitting here like an idiot eating courgette stir-fry.

* * *

I think of how often as women we say 'I hate my body' but I didn't know hate like this until now. I despise it for how it looks, what it's doing. I can't trust it any more after all this betrayal and humiliation. I bargain with a god I don't believe in that I'll be happy with muffin-top hips, stretch marks and moles that have teeny-weeny hairs coming out of them. I will take them *all* and never complain again. Just let me have my old body back.

* * *

I'm off the drugs now, and gradually my weight goes down, but it takes longer than I'd like and I'm still bigger than before. Now my abdomen just looks swollen. Ironically, I look three months pregnant and if I don't dress around this lumpy tummy, waiters raise their eyebrows when I order an alcoholic drink and fellow travellers on the Tube offer me their seat. (I usually take the seat to be honest, it's always nice to take a load off.)

THINGS I KNOW NOW

- Negative feelings about your appearance can manifest in a further distancing from your body; try to remember the good bits, the working bits, the bits you like.

- Invest in your body and appearance: little things like a new nail varnish, haircut, face mask. Even five minutes a day of small acts of self-care can boost your mood and contribute to your happiness.

- It's very difficult to come to terms with the physical changes that might come with this condition or the treatments you take to manage it, and this is a very personal part of living with endometriosis. I will not pretend I have resolved this myself either, but I have learnt that over time a sort of acceptance about how you look is possible if you *feel* well.

- Low self-esteem and feeling like you don't look or feel like yourself can have a huge impact on your mental health and day-to-day mood. Try to get support for this if it is affecting you a lot, talking about it and getting control over the feelings can be a significant step forward.

The Endometriosis Wardrobe, Part two: how to get comfy without 'giving in' (I draw the line at a onesie)

Comfort doesn't have to be unstylish, pyjamas or just anything baggy, but there is a knack to getting it right. Always try to get dressed, even if it's just into some other loose clothes, you'll feel better mentally.

Anything that digs into or is tight around your abdomen can be very uncomfortable if the pain is bad or you're in the later stages of recovery from surgery.

- **Boyfriend and high-waisted jeans**: less pressure on your lower abdomen.
- **A vest top one size smaller than usual**: it sort of holds you, extremely useful for abdominal pain.
- **Maternity jeans and trousers**: these are amazing and no one will know you're wearing them. It means you can have a tight fit on the legs while getting the flexible band around your tummy. (The irony of suggesting these to manage a condition that might affect fertility is not lost on me, but when you try them, you won't care.)
- **Tights and leggings**: hold you gently but are stretchy enough not to compress.

But I want to wear something tight
Sometimes you want something that's tight because it holds you, cradles the swollen and sore bit (like you do with your hands when no one is about). This is when you need:

- **A waist-trainer or a body-shaper**: the kind of thing used to hold your tummy in when you're wearing a very tight dress. Stretchy but tight and worn under clothes – so no one will know!
- TIP: also very helpful for activities when you're stretching your abdominal muscles: dancing, vacuuming, standing for long lengths of time.

Parties and pain

It's hard to go to a party or a wedding on a bad day; your heart may want to go but the rest of your body just wants to curl up and sleep. Here are some tips if you're going to go regardless:

- **Avoid high heels**: the leaning puts pressure on the abdomen and lower back, making it harder to walk and stand.
- **If you *do* wear heels**: stick to a very small heel, platform or wedge so your foot isn't as arched – this reduces pressure on the abdomen. Balance is also easier (especially helpful if you're taking heavy pain meds).
- **Loose tops and dresses**: holding yourself in or worrying about flab is a hassle you don't need, and tense or clenched muscles can make the pain worse.
- **Good support knickers**: so you don't spend the night worrying about looking bloated.
- **Maxi dresses are always welcome**: the shape is flattering if your abdomen is bloated and sore. Cut off some leggings to make shorts if your thighs are rubbing together (they hold your tummy too).

Have an emergency outfit ready to go

Everyone has days when it feels like we have nothing to wear, but if you have endometriosis and you're already pushing yourself this can be the difference between going out or not.

Have an outfit ready that makes you feel fabulous, whatever you're feeling inside.

Little pills (age 27)

My body is under attack from drugs: neuropathic and opiate painkillers, hormone treatments – you name it. My brain slows down. I can't think of words and my speech is slurry. I become distracted, confused and my brain goes wandering on existential tangents. The more bunged up with medication I become, the harder it gets.

* * *

I'm forgetful, making lists and reminders and double-checking everything. People say 'My brain is like a sieve' but mine is more of a colander. I *have* the thoughts and the words but when I go to speak, they've trickled away. I'm used to thinking fast; it's how I write, speak and perform. These are skills required for a comedian but they are also part of my identity. Now this disease is affecting my brain too. When I ask the doctors about this side effect they look at me like I'm crazy – that's the thing, I *feel* crazy. They suggest I try some

CBT (cognitive behavioural therapy) and assure me the right combination of drugs will show itself soon, but I fear there is no version where I get my brain *and* my body back. I try to joke that it's like the *Little Mermaid*, that I have to choose my voice or my legs. 'Perhaps you'll get used to them?' This is all very well but what do I do in the meantime?

* * *

I start to speak less. I occasionally tell close friends when I can't think of the word or I've forgotten what we're talking about. It frightens me and reminds me of how people describe the early stages of dementia. The more conscious I become of it, the worse the anxiety gets. I just want to go home and not see anyone.

* * *

I'm telling my friend Tom a story and the words stop coming out. I stand with my mouth open, waiting. Why can't I remember the punchline? I knew it just a second ago. We develop a game called 'tramadol charades' to help me get to the thought that is lost somewhere in my head, one word at a time, at least we're laughing.

* * *

I meet my friend Heather, a speech and language therapist, for lunch. She tells me it's very likely this is a side effect of the medications; the painkillers and pain slow down the synapse response between my brain and mouth, but it also means there are a lot of messages waiting all at once and some get lost. It's called sensory overload.

She teaches me some strategies to overcome it; slow down, think about what it is you want to say before you start. Recognise the context: does it make you anxious, nervous, relaxed, happy? Then she asks if it happens when I sing or do another voice? Almost the kind of question you might ask someone with a stutter. I try performing for myself that night and find it easier to speak in other voices or sing. So I can improvise as characters to make my friends laugh but if you put me in a situation where I'm with strangers or trying to impress someone I fancy, my speech goes to pieces. I gabble, get very hot, lose all the words and come across as a bumbling fool. Over time it gets easier. I slow down and try not to panic. I contribute less in conversations but my anxiety eases and when I come off the medications it gets substantially better. And now I can even make the words work a bit on tramadol. Who'd have thought it?

13
Explaining pain

If I ignore it, maybe it'll go away?

I coped by ignoring and resisting pain for many years; a few cells in the wrong place would not stop me from doing what I wanted to do. I got on with what I could, when I could, pushing through the not-so-good days and sleeping off the really bad ones. I went to university and when I couldn't stay because of ill health, I switched to one nearer home. When I couldn't perform, I wrote instead. When I graduated I overlooked the limitations of my body, set up Lady Garden and became a professional comedian.

I developed a strong capacity to use mind over matter to keep going and in turn I began to ignore my body. This powerful strategy got me through for a long time. I went to parties dosed up and used the adrenaline of performing to override the pain. I toured and performed and thrashed my body. I was in my twenties and having a wonderful time; I drank and smoked and didn't sleep enough; I stayed up too late and drank large quantities of coffee; I slept on sofas and sometimes didn't go to bed at all. I was a pretty bad patient. While I was always conscious I had a condition that needed to be managed, I wouldn't let it dictate my life. I often laid down in rehearsals, floated around theatres, TV sets and backrooms of pubs all up in my head but apart from having to take breaks for surgeries and various treatments, largely I was able to pretend I was like everyone else. It's incredible what our bodies can endure and what we're able to achieve even in extraordinary circumstances.

I'm not really here (age 28)

I'm doing my first solo comedy show at the Edinburgh Festival. The premise is that my character, Bev, a bleach-blonde, slightly delusional Yorkshire-woman with aspirations of becoming famous, is up here for her big break. The show is ambitious: deliberately fragmented, non-linear and, as farce has to be, intricately structured. This isn't a performance I can phone in and it's the first time I'm doing an hour-long show without five other women to lean on if it's a bad day. The symptoms have been getting worse over the last few months and I haven't had surgery for two years. I've been working full-time in an office job and previewing the show in the evenings, so I arrive in Edinburgh already riding a wave of adrenaline.

* * *

I've done eighteen shows over sixteen days and I haven't taken a painkiller (not even a paracetamol) for twenty. I'm not quite sure how I'm doing this but I am tired, not just festival tired but endometriosis tired. Today the pain is so bad I just cried all the way from my flat to the theatre. But

Explaining pain

Bev doesn't have endometriosis; she is carefree and full of fun. She's agile and sexy; she wears stiletto heels and skin-tight leopard-print clothes. Bev doesn't stop for anyone or anything; she is determined and fierce. I'm going to take a leaf out of her book. I have friends and television producers in and I'm sold out tonight. The show must go on. Eleanor 1 – Endometriosis 0.

* * *

On stage the lights seem brighter and I feel more distant than usual, like I'm not really here. It's vital in live comedy to be very 'present' in the room, especially in stand-up where you have to connect with the audience or it won't work. It's strange, as a performer, to be so conscious of your body while trying to pretend you're in someone else's, but I'm reminded of actors who are able to finish a show with broken bones only to collapse at the end – it's called Doctor Theatre isn't it? Just do that then. But what if the pain becomes so powerful it takes up all my brain and I simply stop talking? Or I can't control my functions? Am I going to shit myself or pass out in front of all these people? They've not paid for *that* kind of laugh.

* * *

Somewhere in the middle of the show I have an out-of-body experience where I'm sort of above my body looking down on myself still performing and the audience laughing (thank God). Maybe I'm dead? This is how it happens in films, right? The world carries on while you float around watching from above? It's like there are three people inside me, three monologues going on at once.

BEV	ME	PAIN
(Actually speaking monologue)	(Calming brain monologue)	(Physical body monologue)
These are actually questions from a session I did back in 2005 when I was a sex worker for the Sheffield City Council. Now I don't know if you're familiar with the statistics but the teenage pregnancy rates had hit the roof and they said to me, 'Bev, can you go in and show them what's what and what's not?' And I said – OK.	These lights are so bright, I can't see if there's a man on the front row, I need a man for the next bit to work. (Shhhhh pain! I'm trying to work.) Wow that's sharp, oooooo breathe, just keep breathing, ignore the pain, Bev isn't in pain. You have to keep going.	Rumble rumble. Stab, twist, sharp. Stab stab, squeeze. POW! Take that! Stab, bang, twist. Ahhhhhhhhhh, stab stab, nausea.
[Hand box to man in front row]	Lean back and slow down, this is a bit where you can breathe, the pace can ease up	You're gonna be sick, nausea nausea nausea.
If you could just have a rummage around in my box please, sir – thank you! It's childish!	Keep breathing.	Stab stab, I'm gonna stab you . . .

Then I am back in my body. I feel as though I've just jumped over an intense wave of pain and now I'm on the other side, still in pain but relieved. Thank God it's over. But then comes the panic, is this going to happen again? What if I don't make it to the end of the show? And then the criticism: it was irresponsible to attempt to do this given your condition wasn't it? What did you think would happen?

* * *

I finish the show but I can't remember it *at all*. My comedian friends assure me my timing wasn't off and the TV producers want to buy me a drink – that's a good sign. As I take off the wig and costume, I wonder what just happened. Maybe I've become a genius user of the mind-over-matter technique? Maybe I've developed superpowers? 'EndoWoman at your service: fighting pain and keeping on keeping on.' God, I hope it doesn't happen again tomorrow though.

THINGS I KNOW NOW

- Mind over matter is a great technique to be able to use, especially with flare-ups, but this heightened state isn't sustainable long term.

- It can develop into a cycle of crashing post-adrenaline and cause more pain 'spikes' and prolonged flare-ups.

- It puts too much pressure on the other systems in your body (e.g. adrenal) which can then affect other functions: sleep, digestion, concentration.

It's a pain in the . . .

Pain can be one of the most challenging symptoms to manage with endometriosis, but until recently I didn't know that *understanding* pain and knowing what is actually *happening* in your body can help give you some control and make you calmer during flare-ups. It's similar to the relief you feel when someone tells you *why* your train is delayed. If you can get your head around it, it will help you to see why certain coping strategies might be more useful for pain than others.

Trying to explain pain pathways and mechanisms is difficult because it's very complicated but there is also still so much we don't know about it yet (this is another area of medicine that needs more research). Trying to make sense of it is made even harder if you're actually *in* pain. So I'm going to try to introduce the basics in more accessible and simple terms, using everything I've learnt from pain sessions, books and doctors. I'm not a medical specialist, more a practitioner of pain, so if this is part of your endometriosis experience (sounds like a theme-park ride) then I urge you to try to understand it and perhaps seek expert support too.

Pain terms and conditions

There are many departments in the brain; they work collaboratively and their messages are so fast you're not even conscious of them happening.

The *amygdala* or '*mid-brain*' is the oldest bit of your brain; it's all about survival and instinct. One pain doctor called it the 'monkey brain' because it's the most primal part of your brain. This is where the initial pain response is received. I think of the amygdala like a reception desk. It decides your immediate response when faced with a threat: fight, flight or freeze.

There isn't a specific 'pain department' so the messages are then sent to multiple parts of the brain for guidance and instruction on what you should do. This includes memories and prior experiences. If we know the pain from before or needed help last time, our brain recognises this and instructs accordingly.

The intensity of the pain is also affected by your emotional response: panic, anxiety, feelings of hopelessness or depression will increase it. Annoying isn't it? The normal responses anyone would have to being in acute or persistent pain are the very things that are making it worse. But if we can explain and understand the pain and why it's happening, despite not liking it, we can calm down this 'threat' response.

It's all in your head

This doesn't mean that the pain is psychological or that you're making it up; it refers to how pain mechanisms work.

Pain *is* in the brain but it isn't in your imagination, it *is* real. The sensory receptors in the area that is injured send a message up through the central nervous system (CNS) to the brain where the sensation of pain is registered, processed and perceived.

Like everything we do, whether it be walking or seeing, the messages are unconscious and being delivered at great speed so the brain can make sense of what action to take. When we *feel* pain, such as when we touch a hot stove, sensory receptors in our skin send a message via nerve fibres to the spinal cord and brain-stem and into the brain.

So although the pain is in a specific area, it is the brain that decides what the pain is and how you should react. So next time someone says 'It's all in your head' you can inform them that it is, but not in the way they think.

Pain remembers

Imagine your brain is a map. It has all of your experiences, beliefs, fears and pleasures written out. Your responses to the world – emotional, psychological, rational and irrational – are based on these experiences, beliefs and knowledge. Pain is part of this. From a young age we learn that pain is a sign that something is wrong; it's a warning to pay attention because you might be damaging yourself. The brain assesses what to do and if nothing is bleeding, broken or in danger, then it will tell your CNS it's OK and the pain decreases.

This is where pain memory comes in. If we know what the pain is caused by and that it's not a 'threat', our brain reduces the pain because it recognises it. For example, the brain knows that period pain isn't a danger so it calms the CNS pain response. But if the pain gets more intense, then the pain pathways start up again and there may be a more panicked response from the brain wondering what is wrong.

THINGS I KNOW NOW

Pain isn't *always* a warning that something is wrong, sometimes this amazing system can get confused – this is referred to as 'chronic' pain. But if the pain gets worse, because something is more serious (like an ovarian cyst), the signals are strong enough to override and break through painkillers, warning you that there is an urgent issue that needs attention.

Bodies are amazing aren't they? (Even when they're being horrid.)

There's another layer of complexity when someone has endometriosis because our period pain is actually associated with a disease, therefore there *is* something wrong. Over time the pelvis has experienced lots of distress, inflammation and pain and the signals can sometimes go wrong, telling the brain there is a danger even when there isn't. These signals can get stronger and more intense over time, the more the pain occurs. One doctor described it like this: the brain has a guard dog whose job it is to receive and assess the pain signals, but when you've experienced trauma in one area repeatedly, the dog can get confused and keep announcing 'Fire! Fire!' These pain signals are sort of useless as a warning because there isn't a 'threat', but the dog has got confused, gone into overdrive. This is sometimes referred to as 'persistent pain' but I'll go into this more later (page 200).

THINGS I KNOW NOW

- It's important to get control of pain early so the signals don't go into overdrive and overwhelm your system.

- This also helps to explain why your coping strategies or analgesic support might need to adapt or increase over time.

If I can't see it, it's not real

Because we are taught that pain is a way of your body telling you something is wrong, it can be very confusing if you're told that all visible disease has been removed, you are now apparently disease-free and yet you're still experiencing pain.

Pain from endometriosis is not necessarily connected to visible disease, quantity of disease or whether all the disease has been sufficiently removed. It can be about how your nerves and CNS respond to scar tissue, adhesions and how long the pain signals have been reacting and on high alert for (this is sometimes referred to as 'neuropathic pain'). Therefore pain from endometriosis may not be explained by a physicalisation of the disease. As we know, the amount of disease has no bearing on the pain someone might feel, which also adds to the difficulty doctors have in explaining *why* you have pain.

Approaching pain

Your approach to pain and how you manage it is shaped by: previous experience, beliefs, associations and traumas that have formed over your lifetime. It can also be influenced by how you were taught to react to it. For example, when you fell off a climbing frame and grazed your knee as a child, did your parents panic? Or did they encourage you to be brave and kiss it better? Did they dismiss it and say nothing was wrong? Did they make you feel silly for being upset? Did they have strong opinions on whether you should or shouldn't take pain medications? These attitudes inform your adult relationship to pain. Similarly, if you are culturally encouraged to think it is normal to have pain, then you're more unlikely to mention it to a doctor. This might explain why it takes some of us years to go to the doctor for pain associated with periods because we are conditioned to think this is a 'normal' part of being a woman.

How's the pain 1–10?

Have you ever been asked to number your pain between one and ten, ten being the highest? This helps doctors get an insight into your pain levels, but it can also help you too, focusing on it gives you some control and helps to reduce the panic.

The flaw in this assessment scale is it depends on when you're asked to assess the pain. I might be yet to experience a worse pain, so how reliable is my ten? My current pain may feel like a ten but it is only based on my experiences so far; your markers change over time. The pain I experienced as a young woman with no pain relief felt like a ten at the time, but since then I have built up a higher tolerance, so that earlier pain might now only be a five compared to the worst days I have now. For example; have you had a really bad pain experience? Childbirth? An ovarian cyst bursting? A broken leg? These things affect your pain responses and how you perceive pain after that event. Pain is also subjective; you might describe it as agony, but to someone else it's mild uterine cramps. Another confusing thing is that some women with endo-metriosis don't experience much or any pain at all, regardless of how much disease they have.

For some people being able to compare and put the pain into context can be very valuable, helping to calm down the 'threat' response, but for others a fixation on scoring their pain throughout the day may in fact heighten the pain response, as their 'monkey brain' will be responding to the pain messages constantly – this is where distractions can be useful.

How do we know it hurts?

Trying to explain and measure the pain you're feeling is difficult while it's actually happening but it's especially hard when it can't be attributed to something we can *see*. There is a general consensus about pain levels: a headache isn't as bad as a migraine, a sprain isn't as bad as a break, normal flu isn't as bad as man flu. But who decides that some pain is manageable and some isn't, especially if they aren't experiencing it themselves?

We are conditioned to assume something we can see is more painful than something we can't. If a bone is visibly broken we can explain the pain, if someone has a cut that's bleeding we assume it hurts, but what happens when we can't see the cause of the pain – like with endometriosis – does that mean the pain is less or doesn't exist? No, but it might make it harder to work out exactly *what* is causing the pain; whether it's disease, inflammation or an over-sensitised pelvic area. Not being able to see the cause can also make it more difficult for the patient to explain the pain and for the medical practitioner to understand and be sympathetic, so it relies on communication – which can be particularly difficult when you're actually *in* pain.

How do we talk about it?

We talk about pain all the time in song lyrics and stories but it's hard to verbalise what physical pain actually *feels* like because we don't all experience pain in the same way. Perhaps the absence of language to describe it is because most people are lucky enough to only experience acute pain a handful of times in their lives, and those who are experiencing it more often, sometimes daily, have quite enough to do without having to make it make sense to the people around them.

But it can really help doctors decipher what might be causing the pain and how they can help if you can communicate what you're feeling, if you can *describe* the pain.

- **Where is it specifically?** Legs, vagina, ovaries, lower abdomen or back, bottom, bowel, rectum, diaphragm?
- **What does it feel like?** Is it intense, itchy, sharp, deep, hot, dull, tender, sore?
- **Compare it to other pain.** Is it mild, moderate, severe, agony, excruciating, acute?
- **What action does it take?** Is it griping, stabbing, shooting, throbbing, aching, nauseating, spasming, winding, squeezing, stinging?

You can start to forget

It's a survival mechanism of the brain to forget the true intensity of the crises but even so I still have some pretty vivid memories. Part of how I cope is to play down the pain, so much so that until I began to write this book I hadn't fully acknowledged that I've lived with pain for twenty-two years. I stopped questioning it because it became the norm. I know I'm not alone, a lot of women with endometriosis experience this but we don't talk about what it's really like, how hard it is to get used to it, to push past it. How we unconsciously factor it into our plans and the energy required to manage it within our busy lives. Will there be time to get the last train without rushing, which will cause a 'spike'. Can we afford a taxi if we

---

miss it? It's like having a very small child or an elderly relative with us most of the time. Pain needs to be considered and looked after, and it's exhausting. No wonder we feel tired.

It will stop

Knowing this helps me to feel I can go on in the hardest, more hopeless moments. It will pass. As my dad always says: 'Nothing stays the same; good or bad.' Over time you will become skilled at handling pain most people would be unable to tolerate, and even if it gets worse than this, you can still somehow survive the next crisis. Remember you are stronger and more capable than you think – you *will* get through it. But you don't win anything for suffering without help or medication and it won't help the pain signals long term to let it run amok. Get support when you need it.

'Chronic' vs 'Acute'

Once the condition has continued for longer than six months they start to call it 'chronic'. I don't like this word, it sounds defeated, nasal and miserable. It feels as if they're describing how patients with chronic conditions become. I prefer 'persistent' or 'long-term', they feel less negative and more hopeful.

Pain like this doesn't begin with a combustible moment, it builds up over time, and you become capable of handling levels that you couldn't have imagined. It creeps up on you and, before your realise it, it's there all the time. I am reminded of the words in Margaret Atwood's *The Handmaids Tale*: 'Nothing changes instantaneously; in a gradually heating bathtub you'd be boiled to death before you knew it.' That's how it feels when everything starts to go with a long-term illness: your muscles, your bones, your skin and hair, bowels and stomach acid; your body feels as if it's disintegrating in increments until you can't remember feeling well at all. It begins to shape your soul and how you feel about everything. I got so used to feeling unwell that all the new symptoms and increasing pain just got swallowed up in it. I stop caring about or expecting anything from my body. I saw it as weak and broken.

Determination, bloody-mindedness (no pun intended) and adrenaline had worked for me for a long time, but a few days after I got back from Edinburgh I collapsed. For real this time, and for longer than a few days. After eleven years of this attitude, I had burnt myself out. I pushed my body too far, asked it to do something really full-on and it didn't like it. It went on strike. I was about to find out that this get-up-and-go approach wasn't a great idea, you need balance. It had meant I could become a successful comedian and have some swell times when it *was* working, so that was a plus. But . . .

That's chronic pelvic pain that is (age 31)

I go to see endometriosis specialists and pain doctors who explain that I now have 'chronic pelvic pain'. This isn't *instead* of endometriosis, it's *as well* as. This is neuropathic pain, a harsh outcome of the disease, trauma and surgeries for so many years. But I'm finding it very difficult to get my head around the idea that the pain isn't coming from new disease, adhesions and scar tissue; that the nerves are broken now too. I'm also strangely irritated. This new diagnosis somehow invalidates my membership of the 'endometriosis club', which is ridiculous because I didn't really want to be a member in the first place. But mostly I don't want to have to learn about another condition I don't understand. I'm already at the endo-my-tether.

A crash course in chronic pain

- The pain system works with the threat system (fight/flight/freeze). For example, if I burn my hand on a kettle, the threat system releases stress hormones within nanoseconds, which increases the pain and I take my hand away.
- It's an incredible system built so you can survive – but when you have 'chronic' pain this system backfires and is unable to differentiate between the 'threat' and excruciating, but 'non-threatening' persistent pain.
- If the pain signals have become repetitive, persistent and powerful sometimes the system can go wrong and your CNS responds to *everything* as a 'threat', even if there isn't something urgent happening. It's sort of stuck in 'fight' mode.
- Your body can then become over-sensitive and you need to find ways to 'dampen down' the pain signals and regulate your system.
- How you perceive the pain is a very significant part of living with persistent pain. If we believe the doctors have missed

something, or don't trust that something isn't really wrong, then the amygdala (or 'monkey brain') will keep firing threat signals – it's not 'the monkey's' fault, that's what it was designed to do.

- Having a better understanding of your condition and situation – i.e. why the pain is there – that this is not new disease, but nerve damage- then the 'logical' part of your brain can regulate the 'monkey brain' and calm down the 'threat' signals.
- This is why 'acceptance' and pain management strategies are important; if we fight and resist the pain, and focus on what we're losing or have lost and compare ourselves to how we were the 'monkey brain' experiences these things as a threat and it begins the vicious cycle again.
- Fortunately, there are things that can be done to get the amygdala to differentiate to some extent, and this can 'turn down the volume' of the pain signals.

Recognising what aggravates the pain and working out how to calm your system down is a major part of handling this diagnosis. Anything that soothes and calms your body will help re-regulate your system: focus on breathing, distractions that bring joy, comfort, relaxation like baths or heat, mindfulness, meditation and pain management techniques such as pacing (see page 204) may also be useful.

This is a complex diagnosis and one that's hard to come to terms with. Speak to your doctor about the best way they can help medically: referral to a pelvic-pain specialist, what medication might help you, psychological and physiotherapy support.

Colleague (age 31)

I'm seeing a pain psychologist. I explain that I've been coping by using mind over matter; that this model of activity and collapse is the only way I know how to deal with this stupid body. But why isn't it working any more? He has a kind face and speaks softly.

DR J: It's got you a long way, I'm surprised it's lasted this long, but it's not going to work any more. The pain signals have become confused and too strong so you won't be able to just ignore it. You've got to face it head on and find new coping strategies. You have to learn to live with it not fight it. I tell him my body and I are estranged, we sleep in separate rooms, I cannot bear the sight of it and we have nothing in common any more. I want to go out dancing and my body wants to lie on the sofa. I want to stand up on stage and make people laugh and my body wants to loll about. I don't know how I'm supposed to find compassion and forgiveness for something that is reducing my life so much?

DR J: If your friend was feeling how you feel what would you say to them?

ME: I'd tell them to be kind to themselves, they're poorly. Have some nice and nourishing food, get comfy under a duvet, watch something funny. Try not to feel guilty, take care of yourself and give yourself a break. You're ill.

DR J: So why aren't you doing this for yourself?

Explaining pain

ME: Because I can't do that *every* day, *every* time this happens. I can't stop to be ill all the time. I'm wasting my life.

DR J: *Try to think of the pain as a colleague you don't like but you have to do a project with. You need to learn to work together.*

ME: I would have left this job years ago if I had to work with this asshole!

He smiles. I tell him that I *know* endometriosis. It isn't reasonable, it's a righteous, egotistical maniac that shows up whenever it pleases, demanding attention and if you give it room, if you listen, it will wail and cry and thump around your body like a toddler in a tantrum. He explains that chronic pain is different to acute, that mind over matter won't work now, that I have to find a way to live alongside it, and that raging against it is a waste of my much-needed energy. Having a mental and physical tug of war will make it all worse.

OK, but what do I do now? It's hard to accept that fighting against the pain is the wrong approach. I don't know how to *live* with endometriosis without being angry with it and resisting it. I am stubborn and unwavering. There are many great women who have had this, it didn't destroy their lives and it wasn't going to destroy mine. This strategy has enabled me to carry on with my life. I come from a long line of strong, ambitious, working women. We are resourceful in times of difficulty and we keep going, on and on till we drop, things like pain don't stop *us*. How was I going to tell them that this way of doing things wasn't going to work?

Accepting the pain feels like giving in. Then it occurs to

me that this sense of 'being defeated by it' is reinforced by the language that surrounds illness, much of which is based on war metaphors. We talk of 'winning or losing battles', 'fighting back' or 'her fight against', we tell children they're 'brave soldiers' and even women with endometriosis have coined the phrase 'endo-warriors'. The culture of battling illness can give you much-needed mental strength not to give in when you need to fight against a disease, but when it's a long-term condition like endometriosis it can also serve to reinforce the idea that there is a fix we haven't found and that there is an end to this struggle, which can be unhelpful. It also encourages me to see illness as an enemy inside, I view endometriosis as happening *to* me, but not part of me and this increases the distance and anger I feel towards it. I resent my body and chastise it for not 'winning' over this disease, when in fact, given everything it's dealing with, it deserves a medal (see, it's hard to stop using the 'fighting' metaphor once you've started isn't it?)

Pacing

This is a pain-management technique used to help break the cycle of flare-ups and 'spikes' in pain and is often recommended to people with long-term pain issues as a way of calming and retraining the signals within your central nervous system (CNS) and retraining your body. It is the exact opposite of my bull-at-a-gate, do everything and then burn out model. When I first heard about it, I said, 'This sounds *so* miserable. Wouldn't it be easier to fix the signals by putting me in a medically induced coma for a few months?' The answer's no, but at least I made my doctor smile.

Here are the basics:
- The idea is that by slowing down your activity and building it back up you will retrain the pain mechanisms in your CNS so you don't live in 'fight or flight mode' and will re-regulate your brain and body.
- This is not about doing *nothing*. It's about building back up what you can do while in pain, or so that you can manage and monitor your energy and activity to avoid flare-ups.

How do you do it?
- You plan each day to include the amount of activity you can do before the pain 'spikes' and then over time (usually a lot of time) you increase the activity. For example: if standing for five minutes is fine but in the sixth minute you are starting to feel uncomfortable, you need to break the cycle of pain by not standing.
- Over a week or two you might be able to do six minutes or seven without aggravating the pain, and so on.
- It's about balance, patience and realistic goals. It might be less activity than you used to be able to do but as one of the doctors said to me: 'You will always lose if you are competing with that person. That is no longer where you are, but you *will* be able to get back to doing more.'

Fundamentally pacing didn't seem feasible. I was single, in my early thirties and living in London. I couldn't see how I could plan each day in such minute detail when so much of my life was spontaneous and my job had lots of unexpected intense activity and rushing around. Coming to terms with and making adjustments to your life so you can live with persistent pain is very difficult. I resisted the reality of this diagnosis for some time, and it had a big impact on my mental health. I couldn't comprehend how I had got to this point, that there wasn't a quicker, easier solution and that I now had another thing to manage as well as the endometriosis symptoms.

I really tried to make pacing work but what do you do if you have to go to the shops for food as your 'activity build-up' but then you need to cook, and you haven't got the pacing time left on your chart? You break your own rules and mutter that the pain specialists are idiots and have no idea how to live with it in the real world outside of their model skeletons and charts. After several months of trying to make it work, I came to the conclusion that it might be more helpful to view it as a set of instructions that could be adapted. This method taught me some valuable lessons about how to approach pain, manage energy and harness enough fight to get going without aggravating the symptoms. I learnt to listen to my body more and made compromises and concessions. I made weird deals with it: 'If I let you rest for a couple of hours today, if I take it slowly, will you behave and let me go to a party tonight?'

It took a long time to get the balance between doing enough to keep sane and happy and not thrashing myself so much it would begin the go-go-go–crash process I had become used to. But eventually I developed a system that works for me; slowing down and being patient enables me to achieve more on the bad days than I used to. This version of pacing has given me a sense of control which means I'm less likely to panic (and make the pain worse), it's also made me more conscious of what might cause a 'spike' and I'm able to recognise the trigger signs quicker. I have strategies in place to calm my body if I've done too much now too (usually a combination of breathing techniques, meditation, lying down and gentle stretches). Even on the days where the pain knocks me out, understanding and working alongside it rather than getting angry and resisting it makes it all so much easier. And the deals I make with my body still sort of work, as mad as it feels do this.

If you can't change something – what do you do next?

I couldn't understand how, even after seeing all the clinicians possible and thousands of pounds' worth of treatment, somehow I felt worse than ever. After a *lot* of therapy, tears, resistance and despair, I learnt that trying to *change* the situation is futile, but your approach and expectations are what change over time. I have also learnt that acceptance and giving up are different things. Accepting that this is the situation *at the moment*, and trying your best not to let it control your life might be enough. We have an extraordinary ability to adapt and acceptance doesn't preclude you exploring new coping strategies or more tolerable treatments; it doesn't stop you from trying to do things even on the harder days. Recognising that this is how something is right now but maybe not forever helps to reduce anxiety and allows you to focus on what can be done about it *now*?

THINGS I KNOW NOW

I know this can be hard to hear, because you still want someone to *fix* this. Put the book down for a bit and go and do something nice. I promise this becomes easier over time.

14
Managing pain

Pills, pills, pills

During the first seven years of my periods I didn't take any pain medication, not even paracetamol apart from the few times of crisis I've mentioned. It never occurred to me to take anything and no one suggested it either. I think we all just assumed I had bad periods, bad luck, and there was nothing to be done but endure them. So I just blustered my way though, passing out and carrying on regardless – letting the pain run amok. It turns out that this wasn't a good idea. Pain specialists have now told me that this strategy may well have contributed to the high levels of pain I now experience.

On the days when the pain feels like it will never end and you're trying to handle it, you get desperate and in turn your body is put under unnecessary stress trying to manage it without analgesic (pain medication) support. Pain is made worse by anxiety, so if it feels like it will never end, and the basic pain medications aren't touching the sides, you begin to panic and this will aggravate the pain further. If you can dampen the pain signals with painkillers, it gives your body some respite and a chance to rest and recover.

It is not uncommon to try lots of different medications until you find the right combination for you. Even the doctors call it a cocktail of drugs, though I've never had a more unpleasant cocktail, and I know which I'd prefer to spend my time trying. Analgesics are likely to be in addition to hormonal treatments and this can mean you have some more side effects to contend with.

THINGS I KNOW NOW

- It might help to ask:

   ∇ What aggravates the pain?
   ∇ What might help the pain other than drugs? (Heat, position, etc.)
   ∇ Are there better times of day to take them for maximum effect and fewest side effects? (E.g. at bedtime if they make you drowsy.)
   ∇ How much can I do without medication?

- If the pain meds are not working or the side effects are intolerable, go back to your doctor and ask if there is something else or a lower or higher dosage? Do certain drugs work better together or at particular times of the day or month?

- What meds do they think will be most helpful for *you* and *your* pain? TIP: Ask about side effects: can you drive, concentrate, drink alcohol on them?

- Long-term use of strong painkillers can cause heartburn, indigestion or acid reflux. Ask your doctor for a PPI (proton-pump inhibitor) drug, such as omeprazole, to help with these symptoms.

- If you're not getting enough or the right support from your GP it might be worth seeing a pain specialist, ideally someone with an understanding of pelvic pain.

Madly, given the number of women suffering, there aren't any painkillers licensed for endometriosis, nor have any been tested for this condition as such, but I asked pelvic-pain specialist Katy Vincent what pain relief might work best for endometriosis-related pain:

There are medications that biologically damp down the pain pathways; paracetamol probably works in the central nervous system, NSAIDs [non-steroidal anti-inflammatory drugs] like ibuprofen or Voltarol probably work by damping down inflammation in the periphery, stopping that drive from irritating the nerves to send its signal out. Opiates work in the brain and probably have some impact on peripheral nerves. Drugs like gabapentin and duloxetine are working in the brain or the brain stem potentially with a bit of efficacy on the peripheral nerves.

'Suppository painkillers? For all the good they've done I might as well have shoved them up my arse!'

In recent years I've found that Voltarol suppositories are brilliant. It's not much fun getting them in (get some lube), but they really help during a flare-up. For many women, the pain is caused by inflammation, so it's worth asking your doctor about NSAID drugs like ibuprofen, naproxen and mefenamic acid. They can be hugely successful and have very few side effects compared to opiates. But be aware that it's not a great idea to take them long-term: do speak to your doctor about this.

THINGS I KNOW NOW

Pick & mix pharmacy

• Always have painkillers in your bag so you don't have to go home during an unexpected flare-up. It gives you flexibility and the freedom to be spontaneous.

• Get rid of the packaging and put them in a nice purse; it helps psychologically, makes you feel less medical and is more discreet, so people are less likely to ask questions when you take stuff.

Pre-planning pain

Having a pain-management plan is crucial for handling flare-ups. It's not only reassuring but it's much less time-consuming to do this in advance, it can reduce the pain in the long run and can help you avoid traumatic emergency situations. I'm not advocating that you pop pills all the time; I'm very conscious of the addictive nature of opiates and that many women find painkillers make them too sleepy or zonked to take regularly. But I *am* suggesting that there is a better way to manage pain than simply trying to get through it without anything. The key is to have the *right* medication. Many women I know self-medicate, regularly cobbling together a medley of over-the-counter pain relief to make it through on the worst days. I don't blame them but there is a better way – speak to your doctor.

Other ways of coping with pain

If you're like me you respond to 'spikes' of pain by trying to stay as still as possible until it passes, with a dry mouth because you're trying not to breathe too deeply in case it makes the pain worse. But there is a big difference between being still and relaxed and being still and tense. In order for it to work you need to unclench, breathe into the pain and try to stay calm.

Why don't you just breathe into it?
'Oh thanks, I'll try that!' I know it's really annoying to suggest something so trivial when the pain is overwhelming, but it really helps. When you're in pain your body can become tense and your breathing shallow and restricted, this is part of the fight/flight response; your body is in survival mode responding to the 'threat'

of pain. Regulating your breath calms down the signals, soothes your system and reduces anxiety, panic and stress, which will lessen the intensity of the 'spike'. It also gives you something to focus on which helps as a distraction technique too.

- Breathe slowly and repetitively into your abdomen – in for three, out for three. In through your nose and out through your mouth. TIP. If breathing out through your mouth makes you feel nauseous, breathe in and out through your nose.
- Try to relax your shoulders and upper body (tight isn't it?).
- Each breath should be deeper and slower than before.
- If you can, lie flat with one hand on your diaphragm and one on your lower abdomen, it helps regulate and calm your body.
- Do it for as long as you need to; you will feel when it's working as your whole body will feel calmer.

Once you get into the habit of doing it, it will become automatic and you will recognise it as an old friend in the worst moments of pain. This strategy has got me to the end of meetings, journeys and performances without completely freaking or passing out from a sudden sharp pain. If you'd have suggested this coping strategy to me even a couple of years ago, I would have laughed at you. But now I use it:

- during flare-ups and with other symptoms like nausea, urgent bowel or bladder pain, feeling faint.
- when I'm struggling to stand for long lengths of time.
- when the pain spikes but I can't stop what I'm doing; I'm driving, at the theatre or cinema, at work or a party.
- when I'm waiting in A&E.

THINGS I KNOW NOW

When the pain is spiking I calmly speak to myself, sometimes out loud. Sort of like you would to reassure someone else when they're panicking. Insane but it works.

▽ Tell yourself it will pass.
▽ You can handle this.
▽ Try not to tense your body. (I know this is really hard in extreme pain.)
▽ Breathe.

Cher-AOKE™

This is one of my more eccentric coping strategies, but I urge you to try it. I originally devised it when I was touring as a comedian and spent a lot of time singing in cars. It turns out every song is more fun if you sing it in the deep, throaty style of Cher. It became known to my friends and I as CherAOKE; like karaoke but . . .

Now I use it on the bad days as a more joyful way of moaning. It helps release frustration, cheers me up and, if I do it really loud, it clears some of the 'endometriosis fog'. Singing also helps regulate your breathing, as you have to dig deep from the bottom of your lungs, so it's a more fun way of focusing on your breath too. You can do CherAOKE alone or with friends, lying on the sofa or in bed, in the shower – it can be done anywhere and, even better – it's free.

Here's how to play:
- The deeper and lower the note the better, so there is reverberation in your chest, like meditative chanting, but more fun.
- It doesn't matter if you are tone-deaf; just sing with abandon, like nobody's listening. Feel the sound from the ends of your toes to the tips of your fingers.
- It works especially well with power ballads but any song will do. Choose something that makes you feel empowered, that's full of *whoomph*. I'm talking your classics: Aretha, Prince, Whitney, Beyoncé, Dolly.

Temperature

You'll already know that warmth soothes pain (you may even have a hot-water bottle pinned to you right now) but did you know that getting too cold can aggravate pain because your body becomes more tense? Or that painkillers can affect circulation, so your hands and feet may be colder than the rest of your body? Get those slippers on!

THINGS I KNOW NOW

You may need wheat bags/hot-water bottles very hot and directly on your body to get relief, but be warned: they can burn the skin, so be careful. Having clothes between the heat and your body helps. Or use electric heat pads that monitor the temperature.

What's the worst that can happen?

Even if your symptoms are manageable most of the time, it's not uncommon to begin to fear they might get worse. Sometimes you might even start to speculate what *could* happen, imagining how you'll handle *that* as well, almost playing out the scenarios in your head like scenes from a film. Instead of looking forward to things you might worry about how you'll cope: what will I do if I forget to pack painkillers, or they run out? What if there isn't a seat, so I have to stand for two hours? What happens if I can't stick to my routine? What if the holiday bed is really uncomfortable and I can't sleep? Then the symptoms will 'spike' and ruin the one thing I'm really looking forward too! This is often referred to as 'catastrophic thinking' and it can lead to high levels of anxiety and exacerbate the very symptoms you are trying to protect yourself from.

THINGS I KNOW NOW

- Being in crisis-management mode isn't sustainable. Negative and overwhelming thoughts contribute to pain levels.

- It's important to try not to catastrophise and remember that this is *one* part of your body and life.

- Mindfulness meditation and talking about your fears can help get this anxious cycle under control and get you back to responding to situations more rationally and healthily.

• Preparing for flare-ups is a good way to get some control over the symptoms but try not to get into unhelpful patterns of pre-empting everything.

The Monkey

Make sure that the schemes you hatch in order to live your life don't *themselves* become limiting. One of the saddest things about this condition is that it can make you preventative; you can avoid certain activities or start to say no to things for fear of not being well enough nearer the time, or because of a misguided concern you'll let people down if you cancel too close to the event. While we may have to consider the symptoms, being overly cautious and conscious of our bodies is no way to live either. As my favourite pain doctor said to me: 'Don't let the monkey ride you.' It can be hard but you have to find a balance between managing the symptoms and not letting them dictate your life.

15
How to handle
a flare-up

Some days we reach for the painkillers because there isn't much choice. They provide relief but they can leave us blurry and unable to do very much. If you know your symptoms are cyclical you can begin to dread these days; worrying how you will get through them, whether they might even be *worse* than you remember. If you're recovering from surgery the endless days can begin to feel like a sort of incarceration, a house arrest of sorts and you can become restless even if you can't do much physically.

We don't really talk about the fact that these days can be very boring too, but over the years I've learnt that *how* you approach them is really important mentally because you still have to fill the time when you're awake. So here are some ideas of how you might survive, and even make use of these days, so you don't go crazy. Sometimes it *has* to be the little things that get you through.

What do I do today?

These days are even more frustrating if there is no structure to them, so one way to get back some control is by making the time useful to you and having pleasurable distractions ready to go. The pain and medications can make you both ethereal and restless so it helps to do things that are distracting without being exerting. It's important to find things that bring you into the present and minimise the despair you may feel that you haven't achieved much today. It also helps to have pastimes that bring the outside, inside when you're stuck in the house as it takes you away from the intensity of the illness for a bit.

What can I do lying or sitting down?

Here are a few suggestions that work for me: reading, knitting, painting, drawing, writing, online shopping, playing games and listening to podcasts, the radio and audiobooks.

Knitting for example has been a joyous addition to my flare-up toolkit in recent years; the methodical and repetitive nature of this hobby is very calming and it's satisfying to have actually created something on these days. It's also a great present producer if you're struggling for money or on a budget; my loved ones have benefited hugely with snoods, hats and mittens and when you get really good you can do it while watching TV too.

Reading

I don't want you to think, while you read my book, that I am not a reader myself, but when the pain is really bad the words are blurry and foreign. I can't make sense of them and I often have to reread the same paragraph over and over, as though trying to commit it to memory, yet I absorb nothing. This usually concludes with me throwing the book across the room. Audiobooks have really helped with this, or sometimes I ask someone to read to me.

THINGS I KNOW NOW

- If something is impossible on days like today don't keep trying, do something else and come back to it later.

- If you see these days as wasted it will only make you more resentful and anxious, which will make the pain levels worse.

- Sometimes you might have to go back to bed. Rest is important but try to mix it up as staying in bed all day can make your mood low.

Aren't We Lucky?

Imagine having endometriosis in the 1800s? If you were rich enough you might have an iron hot-water bottle (mmm cosy) or a maid to mop your brow. You'd be isolated in bed for days, soaking up the blood with old rags and no pain relief. Ignored and dismissed by doctors and your family, made to feel mad and weird. If you were poor I guess you wouldn't have had any of that 'luxury'. You'd have had to go to work regardless, pass out and carry on. I bet this is the first time you've felt relieved to have endometriosis *now* isn't it?

No wonder women with this disease were considered crazy back then: as if the pain and dismissal wasn't enough, some embroidery and an old book for distraction would have sent me over the edge too. There is a lot to be said for getting an iPad for medicinal purposes.

Netflix and ill

During the undiagnosed years I missed a lot of school and one of my main coping strategies was to watch *a lot* of films and TV series. Nowadays there are copious channels, streaming providers and box sets to raid and consume (hooray!), but back then there were only five channels, so I made my way through my brother's enormous VHS collection, and so began my love of film and its ability to inspire and comfort. I could escape somewhere other than the sofa for a couple of hours. I loved films so much I went on to study them at university. There are perks to being stuck on a sofa or in bed – you get to binge-watch like everyone else wishes they could. Even with the best intentions, they're unlikely to be able to squeeze in more than three episodes of an evening and that's by propping up the iPad near the cooker and taking it to the bathroom when they wee. I try to remember this bonus on the harder days.

Watching stuff is my primary coping strategy, the voices and action away from what I'm experiencing work as the best distraction. I am discerning in my choices, the right films or TV can be an amazing source of hope and optimism, but there are some rules.

- **Don't watch mindlessly**: in order to get the true distraction you need to invest in something, be satisfied by the story.

- **Mix it up**: watch a range of things – obscure stuff and popular mainstream, classics and old favourites, films and box sets.
- **Watch your mood**: you learn quickly that films and series that are really poor or particularly harrowing and violent can make you low in mood.
- **Daytime TV**: try not to get sucked into the endless abyss of daytime television; if you watch too much you can end up feeling whizzy and empty, like the viewing equivalent of a McDonald's. Having said that, some morning shows provide easy laughs and entertainment.
- **Help! There's nothing left to watch!** If you use this strategy a lot, this can become a concern. After operation six, I conquered this by breaking my viewing into subcategories. I'd embark on the entire back catalogue of one actor's/director's work: e.g. a Meryl Streep, Viola Davies or a Martin Scorsese Season. Try this or ask friends for recommendations.
- **Ask someone to join you**: the great thing about this coping strategy is you get the pleasure of company, without the pres-sure of interacting. A really great outcome of all my surgeries is the time I've had with my mum when I'm recovering; when I get post-op insomnia we stay up together, watching films into the night.
- **Know when to stop**: I got to a stage where I was watching so much I was confusing it with reality, expecting to see Jon Hamm in the supermarket or wondering how Diane Lockhart was today, as though she were a friend. If you're watching something with subtitles and persuading yourself you're 'reading' it's time to pull the cord.

- TIP: Always consider if this is the best strategy for today, or could you manage something more demanding?

Lists

I love a list. I've always loved them. When you're handling the 'endometriosis fog' or bad days of pain, it's hard to think clearly, sometimes we even forget what might make us feel better. Planning for this time reduces additional anxiety and stress.

A list of why I like a list
- You don't have to keep remembering and clutching things.
- It stops the panic that you've forgotten something.
- Ideas and plans come alive if you write them down.
- It helps you to stick to a budget (which is really useful when you're on heavy medication and easily distracted by a 'cheer-me-up top' or a 'when-I'm-better' pair of earrings).
- It enables you to focus on the present, more joyful things.
- Sometimes just writing the list is enough to get a sense of control.

Here's a list-I-made-earlier list
This is a list of distractions and food made when you feel well, so you don't have to make choices or decisions on the bad days because you already made them when it wasn't as foggy. If doing this feels ridiculous or self-indulgent think of it like a list for someone else you love when they're sick.

- Playlists of music that makes you happy.
- Lists of films or series (Netflix's greatest gift).
- List of quick, easy meals.
- What-makes-me-feel-better list: a nice warm drink, favourite foods, warm blankets and scented candles, essential oils, baths.

I-don't-have-time-for-this-list list

If you're having a bad day but you should be doing something else (work/something fun) it's disappointing, but it can also make you anxious that you don't have time to be ill, that you're missing out or that there will be consequences. This is usually when I start to panic. How will I meet that deadline? I've already called in sick for three days, am I going to lose my job? If I miss today then XYZ might happen. Make a list of what you *really* need to do. Facing it and taking charge alleviates the anxiety and helps you to see what can be put off until tomorrow and if things need to be done today, how you might be able to find a way of doing them.

I'm missing-out list

If you're missing out on something, make a list of things you could do with those people when you're feeling better. It helps with the frustration and disappointment and gives you something to look forward to.

THINGS I KNOW NOW

- Think of things that might help you during a crisis or flare-up ahead of time, so you can just lean back on them in 'emergency mode'.

- Pre-planning makes it easier to cope if you're on your own a lot, but equally if you're lucky enough to have friends, family or a partner to help, these plans will enable them to support you better too.

You can't always 'snap out of it'

We can be harder on ourselves because of the get-on-with-it attitude we're conditioned to have around 'women's problems'. It might help us to get to work or a party, but on *really* bad days such dizzy levels of adrenaline and guilt don't work and when you can't 'snap out of it' you can feel even more defeated by the symptoms. Be kind to yourself: today might be difficult but it will pass, resting isn't conceding defeat, it's about accepting the situation *at this moment*. Try to remember this is one day or a few days where your body needs to stop and recoup.

THINGS I KNOW NOW

- Remember that it's not 'resting' if you are resisting it. If you sit or lie down reluctantly, with anger or irritation, you're using up vital energy and making your body tense.

- The temptation is to eat lots of comfort food and junk, so avoid this by having pre-made or easy stuff in freezer/ fridge.

- Strong tastes are good; the painkillers can make things dull and your appetite reduces on opiate painkillers. Make sure it's something you like.

In the words of Elton John: Don't look at it like it's forever

One of the best pieces of advice I've ever had is: remember the day isn't over yet. You may start to feel better as the day progresses. The pain can subside or change and become more manageable over the day. There will be an end point and you might not have to cancel plans just yet.

It's my vagina and I'll cry if I want to.

It's OK to be upset and not positive all the time. You don't have to always try and look on the bright side. Crying can help release tension and is a perfectly normal response to prolonged pain, disappointment and frustration. You might even feel better letting some of it out.

Don't feel embarrassed of whatever crazy strategies get you through; sometimes I moo into a pillow, once I bit down on my hand until I drew blood. One day I had two long baths sitting on my knees and then curled in a foetal position under a very hot shower. Not only was I the cleanest person in London, but it helped.

The bad patient

I'm not a perfect, Instagram-friendly, fixed-up version of a person with endometriosis. I'm a bad patient sometimes. I eat too late, smoke too much, drink too much, stay up too late, have too much sex, knowing these choices will aggravate the symptoms the next day. Why? Because there is a limit to how much I want to be limited by having endometriosis.

Sometimes I go to a party dosed up, and I drink alcohol, I dance a little (or a lot if I have cracked the timing on the painkillers) and I have a good time. In the back of my mind there is always a voice warning me, 'Well you know what will happen tomorrow'. But I swipe the voice away. 'Not tonight thank you! I'm out on the town and I'm going to have fun for once.' The next day the pain 'spikes' and I crawl around, aching, unable to think clearly and desperate for coffee, sugar, carbs. Was it worth it? Maybe not. But I'm still glad I went. My mental health is better for laughing, for not thinking about this condition for a few hours. And now I have such joy to remember which will keep me going in the harder times.

How to be a bad patient brilliantly

It's not uncommon to become timid or fearful about what might happen when you have a painful or unpredictable condition for some time. 'If I do X it's going to 'spike' the symptoms, and it will be my fault, so I'd best not do it.' Questioning whether something might make you feel worse is a healthy response, but it's important to consider that this might be a pre-emptive reaction because you've been ill for some time; that it is anxiety that is stopping you doing things, rather than the reality of the condition. Could you do *some* of X without doing all of it? For example, at my best friend's hen party everyone went go-karting. I decided it probably wouldn't be a good idea, that it would be too much shock for my body, (it was the right decision, everyone got very bruised.) But so as not to miss out completely I took photos and cheered from the side of the track, which meant I was still part of it.

The worst thing is the self-blame you feel on the days after the activity. You get angry with yourself for overdoing it. The negativity and frustration will exacerbate the pain, so in turn you will be more poorly after doing the stuff you like, then you rage against it and do more anyway and off we go again. Don't beat yourself up for wanting to be 'normal'. Over time you'll learn what aggravates the symptoms, but sometimes you do it anyway because it is worth it for the fun you have.

THINGS I KNOW NOW

- Try to stay spontaneous. Sometimes stay out later than you should. These are the things that will keep you going on the more difficult days. If you say no and deprive yourself of too much you will resent the endometriosis even more.

- You may have to compromise on some things in order to do others.

- It's about balance; a little bit of what you fancy does you good.

- Plan for the day *after* the fun. Remember those lists I talked about?

16
Fertility and endometriosis

When I meet a woman with endometriosis, within minutes they tell me their main concern is their fertility. Mostly they have been terrified by doctors, who are usually not privy to the details of *their* particular disease, nor are they usually endometriosis specialists. My first instinct is to hug them, but I also want to shake whoever it was that made them so stressed and anxious. Endometriosis does *not* automatically affect your fertility; it may increase your chances of having problems conceiving but this depends on where your disease is, what type it is and most importantly your age – the biggest factor for fertility is egg quality. Infertility is not a blanket effect or symptom of endometriosis, but this is not what most women are told when they are diagnosed. It's also not helped by the fact that fertility is often presented as the main issue and doctors tend to talk about this more than any of the other symptoms. It's also the one thing people think they know about the disease, if they have heard of it at all.

Like any woman, we don't know for sure whether we can get pregnant until we try, but even if we're not there yet or the doctors assure us our disease isn't affecting us anatomically, it doesn't stop it being one of our biggest concerns. For many women this is the defining and most worrying part of being diagnosed. It doesn't matter if it will or won't have an impact on our fertility; from the moment someone tells us we have endometriosis we spend much of our lives thinking 'What if?'

Decision (age 17)

They've just told me I have this thing called endometriosis. Then they say something about fertility so I might need to think about having children as soon as possible.

It feels weird to be talking to me about having children when I'm still a child myself. I haven't decided what I'm going to do with my life, let alone who I might be sharing it with, when and where. I can't vote yet or have a credit card. I haven't finished school and I've only just started having sex. It seems as abstract as wondering what job I'll do or what house I will live in when I'm grown up.

Perhaps I should have children now just in case? But I'm not ready, and neither is my boyfriend, and no one knows that it will *definitely* affect my fertility, it might be fine to wait. I'm not changing my entire life for guesswork. So I'm just going to carry on: go to university, try to become a writer and live like any other young woman. But I'm suddenly very conscious of this 'What if?' weight on my back, too aware that the decisions I make now will affect what might be possible later. I start to focus on plans for the future more than before and become very determined to achieve things in a short space of time, with no room for mistakes.

Let's get some advice

I spoke to fertility and endometriosis consultant Michael Dooley and endometriosis consultant specialist Andrew Baxter to try and make some sense of it all.

Does having endometriosis mean I can't get pregnant?
MR DOOLEY: No, definitely not. There may be an increased chance of having problems but it does not mean you cannot get pregnant. Fertility is something that worries everybody, but there's no point, we need to be proactive and see how a) we can prevent the endometriosis getting worse and b) how we can help you conceive naturally or with assistance.

MR BAXTER: It's important to realise that most women with endometriosis can become pregnant – while 5–10 per cent of all women have endometriosis most of these women are still fertile. Endometriosis can reduce fertility and around 35 per cent of women seen in an infertility clinic will have endometriosis. Women with severe endometriosis that affects their tubes and ovaries have a high incidence of fertility problems and may need assisted fertility treatment to help them conceive.

What would you say to women who are worried about this?
MR DOOLEY: We can help you with it. If you're worried, do ask for advice.

MR BAXTER: Although in some cases the disease is persistent, relapsing and resistant to treatment, in most cases fertility can be maintained.

Do I need to have children right now?
MR BAXTER: If women with endometriosis definitely want children they should be advised not to wait any longer than necessary. However, the old advice of being told to 'go away and have your children and then come back and have a hysterectomy' is not appropriate. Having said that, the disease does go quiet during the pregnancy.

Should I look into IVF quicker than most if I'm not conceiving straight away?
MR DOOLEY: IVF almost 'fertilises' disease and I have seen that happen in some women; perhaps they didn't know they even had endometriosis until the treatment has activated it. You have to treat the individual; look at the extent of disease, their age and other parts of their life. Treatment isn't always clear cut. Fertility and endometriosis don't go hand in hand; endometriosis may aggravate your fertility and fertility may aggravate your endometriosis, so we need to look at the individual and find a middle road for them. But solutions can be found for you.

What advice would you give to someone with endometriosis who is trying to get pregnant?
MR DOOLEY: One needs to treat the individual; however I will always talk about good diet. Eat seasonally, think about where it's come from, what processes it's undergone. Keep hydrated. Be careful about alcohol but let's be honest a lot of conceptions happen under a bit of drink – but not too much! Stress itself need not be the problem but it's how you manage it. Sleep is also very important. One of the most important things, I think, is to be happy, positive and romantic, but it's very difficult to hear this or maintain it when you're in a stressful situation trying to conceive. I could tell you to

do twenty things, but you'll get very stressed trying to reach unachievable targets; keep it simple. Everything in moderation, vitamins can be helpful but good diet, an adequate amount of exercise and relaxation must not be forgotten.

How much do we really know about endometriosis and fertility?
MR DOOLEY: I gave a talk recently about the advances in fertility and infertility, and I began by saying we really don't know, and there's so much misinformation, which is not supported by good scientific evidence. We *do* need more research but realistically that may not happen. So, what we need to do is look at the person individually; their age, medical situation, their ethical and emotional beliefs, their financial situation – because sadly not all treatments are available on the NHS. Legal questions may also need to be answered; like donor sperm etc. My job as a fertility expert is to raise all these questions and to help *you* do this with the support and creation of a good team around you. Also – how many children do you want? In some ways my role is also to help you get to your last child, not just your first.

Should I have a fertility MOT?
MR DOOLEY: A full MOT includes a good history of you and appropriate examinations and investigations. However, please don't rush into doing tests until you have considered the implications of what they might show, and this has been fully discussed. Then we can do tests that are relevant to *your* condition. Initial tests could include an AMH blood test (Anti-Mullerian Hormone levels indicate ovarian reserve) and a pelvic, transvaginal scan which would give some idea about your egg reserve but it *doesn't* tell us whether your eggs are healthy, this is age related. For example; if you go to a shop to buy ten tubes of Smarties, you may be

interested about how many are in the tube but I'm only interested in the blue ones because they're the 'good' ones. There isn't a test to check the quality; age is the only factor we can use to guide us. In my opinion the role of the MOT is to help you achieve your own maximum fertility and then maintain it, which could include lifestyle changes. And also please don't forget your partner and consider that they may need to address their lifestyle and have appropriate investigations too.

Should I freeze my eggs?

MR DOOLEY: Egg freezing is worth discussing with your health professional. If you're at risk of significantly decreasing ovarian reserve then you may consider it sooner than other individuals. Again this should be discussed. The statistics of success with egg freezing are improving and the evidence is better than it was a few years ago. The problem though is the process may aggravate the endometriosis. We often need to find that compromise between not 'activating' disease and helping a woman conceive. So I try to see it as treating the *person* not the endometriosis, treating the condition as it presents in that person rather than the general diagnosis.

Should I see a fertility expert as well as an endometriosis specialist?

MR DOOLEY: Try to see someone who is sympathetic and who will treat you as a person not as 'endometriosis'. It's good to see someone who works in a team, which could include surgeons who specialise in endometriosis surgery, experts in scanning and also good counsellors.

Fertility focus

If your fertility *is* affected by endometriosis, it can be a very significicant part of your experience with the disease and I would never wish to undermine the stress and pain that fertility issues can cause. However, it can be frustrating if you are struggling to live with all the other symptoms (bowel problems, repeated surgeries, pain, days lost) if fertility becomes the main focus for the medical system, patients and wider society. It is not uncommon for articles on endometriosis to conclude 'But she was able to have her children'. As if this is the most important triumph over this disease, or that at least it was all *worth* it in some way. This focus on fertility as the main life-altering symptom can undermine the many years we have of just living with the condition and it further excludes and silences the experiences of women for whom even getting out of bed some days is a small miracle in itself.

You may have been told about the possible impact on your fertility because of where your disease is but not want to have children yet; you may be starting to think about it now; you may be thinking of nothing else; or you may not want to have children at all. But it's hard not to get exasperated when the emphasis seems to be on procreating rather than on how you're actually going to live your *own* life with this condition. The feelings around fertility have been one of the hardest emotional issues I've had to manage with endometriosis, particularly in the last few years, and I have found little to support women who are living with this 'What if?' prognosis.

Engine (age 20)

My mother and I have come to see a specialist in fertility and endometriosis. Dr M is a conventional, upper-class gentleman in his fifties; he's charming and has rather taken to my mother (but so does everyone, she's quite something). His kind and perky attitude makes it all feel a little less heavy. He speaks almost entirely in metaphors, a creative flair that feels a bit peculiar alongside his otherwise conservative demeanour but I like it.

DR M: So we won't know whether you can have children until you try. It's very much a case of the pitch looks OK, but are we OK to play referee? I see a lot of women in your situation, they're usually older of course, but what I say to them is what I'm going to say to you; fertility is complicated. Put it like this. I'm looking at a car on a forecourt and it's beautiful, a lovely dark-green colour, nice interior, leather seats, walnut gear stick, CD changer on the steering wheel, big roomy car boot . . .
He's sort of smiling and winking at us. I realise I'm the car. It's certainly a new way of telling me I have a big bottom. It sounds like a line from a rap song, 'Shawty had a big roomy boot'.

DR M: And I'm thinking, I like this, I'll have this. It's expensive, a bit of a treat perhaps, but it's a beautiful car, no one's doubting that.
My mother and I are gripped, a mix of listening intently, trying not to laugh and utter confusion.

DR M: *I'm going to go right ahead and book a test drive, but there's a problem!*
He abruptly raises his index finger.

DR M: *I turn on the ignition – nothing happens – there's no engine! Do you see? There's. No. Engine. In. The. Car. And so the car won't work. It's useless! Looks lovely but doesn't do what it's supposed to. Do you see? Fertility is a lot like that, we simply won't know until you try to 'turn it on'.*
I spend the next ten years wondering if I'm a beautiful vessel with no purpose because my engine won't work.

* * *

In my twenties I became a stand-up comic, toured the country, lived off nothing, had lovers, crap jobs and a wonderful time. But my biological clock was always ticking just that bit louder than the other women I knew and I worried that the disease was spreading or that the multiple surgeries might be making it worse. Fertility didn't become a major concern until I got to my thirties, when all the clocks were ticking anyway. Everyone was having children, my brother, sister, cousins, most of my friends and it didn't seem to be weird to be thinking about it properly now. But I still wasn't in a position to do anything about it.

Fruitcake (age 31)

It's early summer and I'm in a hospital waiting room, a setting that is very familiar, waiting to see a new doctor. Dr H specialises in endometriosis and pelvic pain, he's my fourth opinion. I haven't been to this hospital before but I have been coming to clinics like this since I was seventeen and have come to expect to be the youngest in the room by far. Today though everyone here seems roughly my age. Did I just get older or have 'women's problems' kicked in younger these days? We all sit here pretending to read ancient *Bella* and *Country Life* magazines, occasionally looking around the room and wondering 'What's up with your bits?'

* * *

Forty minutes later Dr H bounds in. 'Miss Thorn?' he barks and looks aimlessly around the room. I smile to indicate it's me but also because this isn't my name.

DR H: Right, so why are you here to see me today?
Here we go again, has he not even skim-read my notes? I am never *not* shocked by this. In what other situation would you start a meeting with someone without giving the impression of not knowing the first thing about them? I'm now going to have to speed through my complex history without taking up the entire appointment. Luckily, while I am so tired of doing this, I have become very good at it. I can reel off the high-lights in a succinct, unemotional tight two mins (comedy lingo for the length of a set in minutes; a tight five or a tight

238

ten). He flicks through the letters in front of him, as if he needs to check I'm telling my own story correctly.

DR H: From these notes it suggests you now have adenomy-osis as well. Is this your understanding?
It's weird how he makes it sound like it's my fault somehow, like I wasn't on top of it, keeping an eye on it and now it's grown here too.

DR H: OK, well. Let's have a look at this . . .
He reaches for a 3D, more fist-size than life-size, plastic model of the female reproductive system. I bristle a little, I don't really like the mini models of organs, they creep me out a bit, espe-cially the way they fall apart. I feel like I'm back in a science lab at school wishing I were better at these subjects than stories.

DR H: So this is what a normal uterus looks like and this is what yours looks like.
He starts to stab the model with a biro pen. I flinch and wonder how many other women have sat though this vivid re-enactment of their disease. The beige model is now covered in black ink spots. It reminds me of the time I drew a moustache on my sister's Barbie doll, thinking it would wipe off. It didn't. His ferocity is alarming but I don't think he's realised this is the only model in the room and he's probably going to need it again to depict some other deficit one of the women sitting outside has. (Unbeknown to her of course; she's just reading *Bella* and wondering what's taking so long.)

DR H: A normal womb should be soft and spongy like a cake—
The comedian in my brain tells me that this is like a

gynaecological episode of *The Great British Bake Off*. Then I remember that this isn't funny. My womb should be soft and spongy and he's about to tell me it isn't.

DR H: —but yours is heavy and solid-like a fruitcake. You're a fruitcake.
I laugh. He's hit the jackpot; a doctor telling a woman with endometriosis that she's mad. He frowns.

DR H: Do you understand?
ME: Yes. I think so.
  I grimace, my laughter fading by the second. WIWIS is: I think you just called me a fruitcake – as in crazy – and that's pretty funny and I'm going to put it in something. Except no one will believe it of course, because it sounds like a script. A funny routine about a doctor who's telling someone it's very unlikely she'll be able to have children and I've put this in to lighten the mood. This didn't happen they'll say, but I'll swear that it did. I sit quietly, looking at him and the now-discarded biro-ed model, while he tells me that my 'window of fertility' is closing rapidly and given I'm single, have I considered a sperm bank? Finally he states that there are 'plenty of bene-fits for single mums', that I'd 'be surprised'. Yes I would. I leave the appointment with the advice that I should start trying to have children immediately or the choice will be taken away from me.

* * *

Within ten minutes everything has changed; this is the first time anyone has said that fertility is *definitely* a problem for me. I wasn't expecting this; I thought I was here to talk about treatments no one else had thought of yet. I wish I'd brought someone with me. I hold it together enough to hand a form to the receptionist and find the toilet. In the cubicle I stuff a wodge of tissues in my mouth to stop the noise. After about five minutes, I gather myself. When I look in the mirror I see I now have two swollen eyes to match my spotted uterus.

Adenomyosis, Meet Endometriosis, I think you'll find you have a lot in common. . .

How do you say it and what is it?
AD-EN-O-MY-O-SIS. The cells of the lining of the womb are found in the muscle wall of the womb.

Who gets it?
Approximately 1 in 10 women have it, it's more common in those aged 40–50 and in women who haven't had children, but it can affect any woman who has periods. It's similar to endometriosis but it *is* a different condition. It's not unusual to have both, but they can occur separately too.

What are the symptoms?
Persistent pelvic pain; a heaviness or swollen abdomen; heavy, painful or irregular periods; pre-menstrual pelvic pain; painful sex or bowel movements; a dragging sensation down thighs and legs. But some women don't have any symptoms.

Sounds pretty similar. How do they diagnose it?
It can't be definitively diagnosed without biopsy of the uterus post-hysterectomy but transvaginal ultrasound or MRI scans are the best ways to evaluate presence of disease without surgery. It can sometimes be misdiagnosed as fibroids (and vice versa).

Could I have prevented it?
No, it's bad luck. It's not contagious and it's not cancerous.

Please tell me we know how to fix this?
Like endometriosis, we don't know much about it, but it's likely that genes, hormones and the immune system are involved. There's no cure but you can manage it. Symptoms usually stop or lessen after menopause.

How do we treat it?
The IUD (coil) or GnRH (can only be used for a limited time though) are effective and can help stop the disease progressing. Hysterectomy is the only way to remove the disease all together, but this comes with other issues to consider. In terms of pain management, NSAIDS such as ibuprofen or naproxen can help and heat pads to ease the cramps.

Does it mean I have a higher risk of infertility now then?
It doesn't necessarily decrease your chances of getting pregnant, but it may increase the risk of miscarriage or premature birth. Speak to your doctor about *your* disease. Hormonal treatments can be timed around your plans or fertility treatments such as IVF.

Reminder (age 31)

Fruitcake-gate was a couple of months ago and since then I have become preoccupied with babies and fertility. I feel foolish that I had hoped it would be OK, that this is *my* fault for waiting. I have a profound sense of loss. It feels like grief. But it seems ridiculous grieving for something I never had and somehow fraudulent to feel sad about something I don't absolutely know I won't be able to do yet. But I *do* know that each day is one more that has passed since the doctor said, 'If this is something you want to do, then you should do it now.' I'm in a limbo place; too conscious of this thing I might not be able to do. But without knowing for sure, I can't give up hope. It's said that there are five stages of grief: denial, anger, bargaining, depression and acceptance. For me grief has never been a linear journey, it's not like climbing a ladder until you reach the end. I feel these emotions simultaneously.

I can't move for babies. I'm suddenly surrounded by them. Magazines emblazoned with 'bump watch' and every film or TV show seems to be about having them, seemingly everyone has a baby carrier on their front. Everything, every-where, seems to be about them.

It's also made harder that 'women's problems' are treated in the same hospital wings as the more joyous parts of what women's bodies can do. In the entrance I walk past brand-new parents and expectant mothers, the birth centres and antenatal care. A cruel reminder of what I may never have and the reason why I'm here is the reason why I won't. I share waiting rooms and have ultrasounds in the same clinics as the women who get to see their babies for the first time but I just see an empty womb, save for cysts and disease. I sit there trying not to catch anyone's eye and wonder what it would be like for these organs of mine to bring joy and love, not just pain, in every sense of the word.

THINGS I KNOW NOW

- **Research and understand your options**: there is strength in knowing what's possible, ignorance breeds fear and worst-case scenarios.

- **Look on the Endometriosis UK website**: they have fantastic information on fertility and pregnancy (see page 342).

- **Recognise triggers**: high-profile baby-watch in the media, baby showers, being around pregnancy and babies. Seeing pregnancy can sometimes be harder than seeing women with children. Perhaps because you can still be a mother, but you might not be able to do the pregnancy bit.

- **Pregnancy announcements can be bittersweet**: you're not a bad person if you feel jealous or sad when someone tells you their joyous news. It doesn't mean you don't love them and their children. You can feel both things at once.

- **Find a way to talk about it with people you trust**: letting them know of this emotional trauma helps them to be more sensitive, aware and understanding.

- **Some people will be more sympathetic than others**: true friends will jump into it with you, fearless, and they'll try to listen and help.

Freezer (age 31)

I've come to see if I should freeze some eggs. The doctor is telling me the results of the FSH blood test, which checks my ovarian reserve; basically how many eggs I have left.

FERTILITY DOCTOR: You have fewer than you should for your age, but nothing to worry about immediately. Perhaps you should freeze some eggs though? The stats aren't great, but think of it as an insurance policy.

But it's not that simple when you have endometriosis; the process to harvest the eggs involves injecting a vast influx of oestrogen and this is likely to aggravate the disease. It feels a bit crazy when I've only just finished a treatment to *suppress* oestrogen and had an eighth surgery to *remove* disease. My hormonal balance feels a bit fragile anyway. Is it a good idea to seesaw my body in the opposite way from desert to flood?

The process is also expensive and then you have to pay to freeze them too. When I first saw the figures my initial thought was, 'Can't I just ask my housemate to shift some of his Quorn out and I'll pop them in my *own* freezer?' No, is the answer.

Well. I can't afford it so I'll just have to wait.

* * *

While researching online I find a clinic offering an egg-sharing scheme. The idea is that a couple who can't conceive fund the egg-boosting and extraction process and in return they have some of my viable eggs. The only bit I pay for is the freezing costs of the ones left over. It seems like a good option: it gives another woman the chance to have a child and reduces the costs hugely for me. I keep scrolling and find something odd – a list of other providers, like a 'Compare the Market' for fertility treatments. It looks like this:

Superdrug	£1,919.22
Asda	£1,171.41
Boots	£1,893.70

Syringes and hospital fees, etc. aren't included of course. Welcome to private medicine. The brazen price packaging of something so sensitive makes me uncomfortable but I'm not surprised. Capitalism will weave itself into anything where there is money to be made, however distasteful it seems to be targeting people at their most vulnerable.

I ring my friend Tom and we laugh at how it's the kind of ridiculous, far-fetched thing I would write a comedy sketch about. I joke that I'll get it done at Boots on a double-points weekend, I have my eye on a perfume. If I go with the supermarket option is it like photo-processing or dry-cleaning

– eggs done in an hour while you wait? Are the cheaper providers using freezers that are less reliable, or do they just sling them in with the fish fingers and chips in the frozen aisle and hope for the best?

But I shouldn't have laughed so soon.

* * *

Six months later and I'm genuinely thinking about doing it now. I go back on the site and find that I'm not an 'acceptable candidate' because I have endometriosis. I phone them for clarity:

RECEPTIONIST: *The concern is your eggs will be damaged. And as endometriosis is genetic, the recipient doesn't want eggs that carry hereditary diseases.*

No one knows either of these things for certain. But surely the women involved in the scheme, both recipient and donor, would understand more than most what such exclusion feels like? I feel so betrayed. I was about to give some of my limited eggs to you: a gift, a treasure, a chance to be mothers too, but you don't want them? Why do you see me as damaged goods? I thought we were all in the same compromised fertility boat here?

As I put the phone down, my whole body feels very heavy; perhaps it's the weight of my heart as I realise even my backup plan has gone up the swanny. To cheer myself up, I get that perfume.

And then I get angry.

* * *

My periods have been appalling from the day they started, but to be told none of this was worth it, that I've been dealing with this shit for twenty years for no reason? All those years spent panicking about unwanted pregnancy, only to find myself panicking that I won't have a wanted one either.

All the money on tampons and towels and paracetamol and new knickers.

All the worry about the right birth control and the side effects.

All the condoms and morning-after pills and anxiety when I was late.

All the mess and the responsibility and hot-water bottles and being kind to myself.

All of this and it was for nothing?

I want it out. Just take it out.

I consider it for a long time but when I ask Dr B for a hysterectomy he tells me he doesn't think it will work for me, that my reaction to the pseudo-menopause is a good indicator of how I would feel and this wouldn't be a reversible treatment. But also there's no way to know if the pain is just caused by disease now, the scar tissue and adhesions and so many surgeries are likely to be part of it too, so it wouldn't help with that. Three other specialists concur. I think I'm just desperate for this pain to stop, rather than really wanting to do this anyway, so I will have to find some other way to live with it.

Facing it time (age 31)

My younger sister is pregnant and we are on FaceTime. She's telling me how uncomfortable she is, that it's affecting her sleep. My eyes sting with tears. It catches me out sometimes, I think I'm fine and then I am acutely aware that I probably won't ever be lucky enough to be uncomfortable because I'm pregnant. My sister and I are incredibly close, we talk about everything; but I'm jealous. I want her to talk to me about it, I want her to share it and to be included in her experience and excitement, but it's also too painful. I move from the camera so she can't see me crying and then make some excuse to hang up.

* * *

My therapist tells me I need to talk to her. But I don't want to be selfish or make this about me. I worry she'll never mention *anything* for fear of upsetting me. I don't want to be excluded from it, or for her not to share her feelings at *all*. That feels even worse. It'll pass I think. I just need to squash it back down. My therapist looks back at me, concerned, this is *not* the way to manage it.

* * *

Two weeks later I'm with my sister in a Mexican restaurant. The sadness smothers me. I shakily find the strength to tell her how I feel, how much I already love my niece and she isn't even here yet, how I want to be part of her pregnancy and motherhood and I don't want her to feel she has to hide things or hold back but it's sort of unbearable for me at the moment too. She cried. I cried. The tacos got cold and wet with tears and we cuddled over her bump. I feel huge relief that I've said something and equally glad they've sat us away from anyone else.

And the best part? Nothing changed. We talk like we always have, but she just asks me how I feel a bit more and is more aware of how I might feel in particularly 'baby' environments. That was all I wanted, she just needed to know.

THINGS I KNOW NOW

Baby showers are hard.

- **Protect yourself and don't feel guilty**: can you handle this right now? Could you go to some of it but not all? Send a gift but don't attend?

- **If you go, confide in one friend**: let them know how difficult this is and maybe have a signal so they can get you out of the conversation/situation if you're struggling. Advocates in real-life situations as well as medical are very useful.

- **Be kind to yourself**: pop out of the room if it becomes overwhelming, or simply leave.

How do we talk about it?

Since the age of twenty-five, people, often ones I barely know, will ask me if I have children, followed swiftly by an array of questions about why I don't – and it's always at weddings or something joyous that dictates I shouldn't cause a scene. It goes a little something like this:

'Do you have children?'
'No, not yet.'
'Do you want to have them?'
'Yes. I'd like to . . .'
'Are you married?'
'No.'
'But you have a boyfriend?'
'No, not at the moment.'

They wince, I smile and they suddenly need a refill. I smile again but it's a different smile, one that recognises the madness of what's just happened. *They* started a conversation, which then made *them* feel uncomfortable, so they exit hastily leaving *me* feeling uncomfortable like it was *me* that brought it up.

It is strange that *any* woman should have to deal with relentless questions about what plans she has for her uterus; it is nobody's business but your own. But if pregnancy is something you cannot do, or even *think* you can't, these probing questions are a deeply upsetting reminder. This is especially distressing in a context where you might be actively trying not to think about it; like weddings and baby showers. It might appear to be a harmless conversation starter, perhaps a way of finding common ground, but you're essentially saying 'sorry do you mind if we talk about your womb?'

If you have a condition where you might have concerns about fertility or even *know* that it is impossible for you to conceive, it is something that can be very painful to discuss at all, with anyone, let alone a complete stranger.

I promise myself that next time I'll be honest. They will rue the day they so nonchalantly bring this up as if they are asking 'Have you tried the salmon?' I want to say that I don't want to talk about it thanks, that this is harder than one question. That I don't know yet and neither do the doctors. I want to be that guy sometimes. But I don't. People who ask this stuff don't know they're dancing about on landmines; they have no idea that I have a lump in my throat and my chest is tight. They just wanted to know if I was like them.

You're just a baby machine

It also occurs to me that these are the automatic questions we ask *all* women when they hit a certain age. Rather than asking about their work or their lives, they become reduced to their marital and maternal status. I would guess people aren't asking the young men in the room such things. There may be questions about his love life or if he's thinking about settling down but it's likely that they will come after a lot of curiosity about his work, where he's living, his holiday plans.

By repeatedly concentrating on babies and romance we are reinforcing the idea that these are the most important things in a woman's life; that women only achieve their full potential once they become mothers and wives, and that whatever else they do is filler before the bigger, 'more meaningful' life events. The fixation on these things means we ignore the value of the women in front of us and diminish the other achievements and joyful parts of their lives. It also assumes that the inevitable ending or dream for *every* woman is having a baby. For some it is, for some it isn't and for some it isn't possible.

It's really important to recognise that all this societal expectation and pressure makes it much harder for women who cannot have children but wanted them. Coming to terms with this is made much more difficult by the perpetuation that a woman's function is to be a mother and that without children she is thought of as 'unfulfilled' or 'not whole'. This is something which is often reinforced in the media, and indeed by these conversations with strangers at parties, and it can make us feel further isolated and excluded from 'the group'.

Everyone's got a solution – handling unhelpful input

If I cautiously tell someone I have endometriosis their first response is usually 'Does that mean you can't have children?' What surprises me most is the carelessness of it, the blunt way I am asked about something so personal. People seem more nervous about asking what I can and can't eat on a wheat-free diet than they are about my uterine status. Maybe they're worried they might *really* upset me if they remind me I can't eat pizza. I wonder if the reason people latch on to this as the 'main' symptom is because it's the most relatable bit that people can talk about (or think they can).

More recently, if I'm strong enough, I try to say, 'I have a condition that is likely to have affected my fertility, so I'd like children, but it might be difficult.' I see the wide-eyed panic; they splutter and start offering advice to make up for their awkwardness. What about IVF? Can't you freeze your eggs? Can you do surrogacy in this country? Could you be a teacher/auntie/godmother/insert any maternal-ish role/job. Why don't you get a dog/cat/rabbit/insert any animal that could be seen as a replacement for a child. These things are suggested in haste because people feel sad or a need to resolve it. But I didn't ask you to.

The 'flippant hysterectomy'

This is often suggested to me: 'If it's causing you this much trouble why don't you just have a hysterectomy?' Like my uterus is a car that is costing me too much to fix so I should just get rid of it. It's quite a strange thing to suggest to a young woman just because you're impatient or out of ideas. I wonder if they would be so flippant if *they* were faced with this 'choice'?

'Why don't you just adopt?'

People who say this are usually unaware of the complexities of adoption, as though it is as simple as going to look at some cats and saying, 'I'll have that nice black fluffy one in the corner please.' I now respond with similar short shrift: 'Yes that is an option, but it's a long process. I'm not sure it's something I can do at the moment but thanks.' What I want to say is: 'If, for one second, you were to imagine life without your children, or grandchildren, that you wouldn't see yourselves in their faces, that they didn't have the famous family dimples, noses and mannerisms – imagine that for a moment, and then you might have an insight into the grief one feels when dealing with this stuff.'

'Why don't you just have a baby?'

This is perhaps one of the hardest suggestions to contend with; the very thing that you are being told is potentially at risk is the thing that is touted as a fix, even by doctors. It's deeply insensitive to suggest this to women who are struggling to conceive or are unable to because their disease is making it impossible. Perhaps the intention is to provide some optimism, but all it does is perpetuate the myth and make women frustrated and sad because this supposed 'solution' for the problem *is part* of the problem.

Why do people do this?

When people offer opinions on something they know nothing about it can be very frustrating and hurtful, but it's usually because they are deflecting their own anxiety or sadness that they can't offer a happier ending. But sometimes situations *are* difficult and they *can't* be resolved. All anyone really needs to say is, 'I'm so sorry you're going through this. If you ever want to talk about it I'm here if you need me.'

For women with endometriosis who are having fertility issues or are unable to conceive, the added cruelty is that the very organs that are causing us such pain (both physically and psychologically) are also the ones that are betraying us once more. Impatient questioning and implied blame does not make this any easier. You need time to get used to the situation, and the feelings that come with it. It's natural to grieve for something you wanted and there is no fixed time frame in which to do it. You may want to look into other ways to have children, but you *must* be allowed to feel these things first, before embarking on another way to do so.

> **THINGS I KNOW NOW**
>
> I used to struggle with these questions and try to appease the discomfort of others. But now I say: 'I would like children, but I have a condition called endometriosis, so I might not be able to. I'll have to wait and see.'
>
> Then I can: walk away/change the subject/educate them, but I'm not obliged to 'fix' it for *them*, explain it or talk any longer than I wish to.
>
> Do whatever works for you.

Hope at the end of the tunnel

Many women I know with endometriosis (and adenomyosis) have had children. Some have needed some assistance, some haven't, some have even stopped trying and then it's happened. Even now my doctors don't actually *know* whether my fertility has been affected so we won't know for sure until he (whoever I finally choose) drops his trousers and we hope for the best. What I have learnt though is that living with a kind of pre-emptive grief for what might be, what might have been, what you can't (maybe) have, is an impossible state to be in. Over time it becomes less raw and doesn't absorb every waking moment. It morphs into a low-level angst that twinges once in a while and with a bit more time it's no longer so completely heart wrenching to talk about it.

I began to share some of what I was feeling with my closest friends, my sister, my mum, all of whom are mothers. I talked to my dad and brother who are both fathers. I sat on a bench in the middle of the V&A with my great aunt and she took my hand and told me about her life without children, that although it was a choice, it also made her sad sometimes. She spoke of other wonderful adventures and the importance of other kinds of love and relationships. And then she said, 'Also, you have smashing breasts and they'll stay like that if you don't have babies. So that's something!' And I laughed and cried and we sat squeezing each other for ages, while people walked around us, presumably thinking one of us was dying. I talked to other women with endometriosis who couldn't have children and found we shared similar feelings, which gave me some comfort and made me feel less alone.

Everyone responded differently but mostly they just listened, and sometimes became more thoughtful. Some people still blunder their way through saying thoughtless things like, 'You wouldn't know, you don't have children.' And while this *never* stops being desperately painful, I have learnt that, mostly, they don't mean to be unkind, it's usually just insensitivity, so I swallow hard and walk away or I challenge it. Most people, and the only ones you should want in your life anyway, are kind and become more conscious of how you might feel, but most importantly, they do this without excluding you from their lives with their children.

Words Matter Here Too

What's with the pejorative terms for women who don't have children?

Childless
Sounds like I'm missing something? It's not as much fun as the other -lesses: painless, paperless, weightless, which are all great things to be.

Child-free
Well I'm not. I have lots of wonderful children in my life – and they aren't free! I love nothing more than choosing the right book, toy or jumper for these beautiful children. And then I wonder if they do some of the clothes in adult sizes, they're right up my street.

17

How do I live with it?

This chapter looks at some of the other things that we might have to manage as part of living with endometriosis; how to cope when the pain becomes too difficult to handle on our own, how to juggle symptoms with work and the financial implications of living with a long-term health condition.

Emergency endometriosis

Women with endometriosis often find themselves in A&E. It's not because we are weak, or opiate addicts, nor are we looking for sympathy or to jump the queue, but if the pain gets worse than we're used to, it can be distressing. We don't ask for help lightly, it's not uncommon to wait for hours, hoping it will ease, but we know when something feels *really* wrong. The medical advice when the pain has increased rapidly, is constant or unmanageable is that it might be indicative of a more urgent issue – like an ovarian cyst. We need to be assessed, have a scan to rule out anything more serious and offered better pain control. So it can be perplexing to be treated dismissively at the hospital when you are only following that advice.

The doctors and nurses in emergency rooms are incredible, handling major traumas day and night, but they are not equipped or trained to deal with a complex, long-term condition like endometriosis. Pain that appears to be unexplainable from the outside tends to be misunderstood, delayed or discharged back to outpatient teams. But the problem is, there isn't anywhere else for us to go when the symptoms change suddenly or the pain becomes impossible to manage on our own and this can be one of the most difficult and frustrating parts of living with endometriosis.

DIY (age 33)

Middle of the night
I wake up with a sudden sharp pain in the left side of my abdomen. I lie in the dark skimming through my options. After years of living with this, I have developed a capacity to be calm and practical at the same time as experiencing acute levels of pain and anxiety. I need to take more painkillers but that will impact how much work I can do tomorrow and I've lost too many days already. I don't have time to have endometriosis, I'm writing a book about endometriosis! But without them I won't get *any* sleep; painkillers it is then.

Morning
Wake up, more drugs, try to sleep again. Can't. Get up, too nauseous to eat, manage two dry oat biscuits. Double up the codeine and tramadol, it takes the edge off. Have a hot bath.

Curl tightly on the sofa. Back to bed. Try to remember it's just a flare-up, it will pass, don't panic. But I *know* pain and this isn't the usual kind.

Midday

On FaceTime my brother tells me I look really ill and need to call a doctor. The GP tells me to go to hospital as soon as possible, he believes it could be a cyst rupturing or twisting – I need a scan. I've had three cysts already, this isn't news to me, but I really don't want to go out into the cold, into clothes, into *another* hospital. While researching this book I've learnt that it's not a good idea to let cysts rupture on their own (which I have every time), and if the pain is extreme, sudden and continuous then it could be ovarian torsion. This is when the ovary twists. It is relatively rare, but it can be more common with cysts. He offers an ambulance but I've read recently that they cost £750 a call-out and I don't want to waste already strained NHS resources. And what if I take an ambulance from someone who is having a heart attack? I'll get an Uber. I remember my bank balance, I can't afford a taxi, can I make it to the train? Try to stand up. No, I won't be walking anywhere. Order taxi, sort budget later. The hospital have my notes and an endometriosis centre – they'll know what to do.

* * *

I've ignored my own advice and come alone. I join a queue, clutching my side as though I'm pushing a hernia back in. I explain as calmly and politely as I can what I think is happening, and that I need to see a gynaecologist as soon as possible. 'You'll be waiting a long time,' she says, as if any of this is a choice. I take a seat.

It's like endometriosis Groundhog Day. I know how it works: I will wait in line like everyone else, eventually a nurse will take some blood and do a urine test for pregnancy, then an on-call gynaecologist will come down and assess me. This might take several hours. They'll tell me not to eat or drink in case I need surgery and I might get some interim medication and a bed if I'm lucky. I drift into another space, somewhere between the conscious and unconscious world, a sort of trance state where I lose track of time and reality. I think this must be the second rung of survival mode: you go past panic and asking for help when no one else is panicking or helping.

Quite worried now though. If this is an urgent issue people aren't being very urgent about it. Every minute I sit out here I might be losing my ovary. I squirm around on the hard plastic seat, one of four connected by a steel bar. It shakes every time someone stands up or sits down, I feel every jolt as people get up to smoke or berate the receptionist. I try to focus on the TV with no sound.

More time later

A doctor ushers me into a cubicle. I writhe around on the chair and try to briefly explain my history. He writes something, it's upside down to me but it looks like 'splenectomy'.

ME: Sorry, what have you just written?

DR: *Splenectomy.*

ME: I haven't had that. Endo-me-trio-sis.

DR: *What is that?*

Wow. Keep breathing, you'll get a scan soon.

ME: Shall I spell it?

DR: *Yes*

I spell it.

ME: Sorry, are you not a gynaecologist?

DR: *No, I'm a GP. So this endo mett-tree-i-tris . . .*

Sweet God.

DR: *I think I remember it from my training. It's ectopic womb tissue isn't it? Can get to lots of parts of the body? And it's a long-term thing, did you know that?*

Err yes, it has come up once or twice.

ME: Yes. I've had it for a long time, that's what the nine operations were for. But as I say the pain is substantially worse
and specifically in my lower left quadrant.

DR: *You seem to know a lot – are you a nurse?*

Why does he assume I'm a nurse not a doctor? Is it because

I'm a woman? (Note to self: this man might not know what he's doing.) He calls the gynae department, getting most of what I've just told him wrong but I'm in too much pain to argue.

DR: You're in a lot of pain, yes?

Finally. Someone has noticed. I'm going to get some meds now. It'll be OK.

DR: They say the worst pain is kidney stones, followed by a shoulder break.

Do they? Do they really? I'm not having a 'pain-off' with you, mate. You're mansplaining pain to *me*? Where are the drugs? I need the drugs! I don't care if I look like an addict now, this has to stop. He sends me to another waiting room.

* * *

Even more time later

The nurses tell me I've been prescribed some Voltarol supposi-tories. I am loath to have fingers up my bottom disrupting my swollen body, but I'm nothing if not desperate. They bicker loudly about who will put them in and finally ask if I would mind doing it myself. They pass me two bullet-shaped capsules, a glove and a sachet of lube. Could I do a urine sample too?

* * *

In the toilet I attempt to wee into a small cup but my aim is all over the place. I'm trying not to waste it, or get it on my hands, but I'm also worried about getting it on the label, which will dissolve my name. ('She dissolved her own name' sounds like the tag line of a thriller novel you buy at the airport when you realise you didn't pack a book.) Then it's suppository time. Now I don't know if you've ever tried to put one in in, but it's not easy. Add into the mix that I can't lie down because I'm in a public toilet and there's a cannula needle in the crease of my right elbow so I can't bend my arm. So here I am twisting and stretching and trying to push them in and I suddenly see my whole body reflected in a large mirror on the wall. (Why is there a large mirror in a toilet?) I laugh, because while this is grim, my God it is funny. Fancy coming to hospital and being given DIY suppositories!

* * *

Back in the cubicle, squeezing my ass together trying to stop my rectum spasming the capsules back out, two young gynaecologists arrive. I repeat my medical history again. The woman writes it down and the man asks stuff. He says he has to do an internal exam. I know it's unnecessary if this is endometriosis related; it will show him nothing more than I am in pain and we know that already. But he insists. It's protocol. I worry he won't send me for a scan if I say no, so I let him do it. I look at the ceiling. Keep breathing. I ask him to stop. The have-a-go gynae paces at the bottom of the bed, shrugging. He's like a teenage boy who has been rejected; annoyed he's been unable to finish the task he seems to feel entitled to do. I half-expect him to kick a chair. Through the tears I apologise that I'm in too much pain for him to complete it. I am appalled that I'm doing this, but

265

when you are vulnerable and at the mercy of someone you do strange things. He looks at the glove with disdain, snapping it off and putting it in the big yellow bin marked 'Toxic waste'. If I didn't feel shame already, I do now.

DR: Well there's nothing of interest on inspection.

What every woman wants to hear when someone has just looked at her vagina. He opens the curtain fully, so the other patients waiting can look in. I pull my legs up to my chest. He returns a few minutes later, his consultant says I need to have a scan immediately, something I have been saying for five hours now.

* * *

That night
Then it gets better. The sonographer was kind and gentle. The scan showed a lot of fluid, perhaps a ruptured cyst, but he tells me my ovaries are mobile. I remember this because I said 'I'm glad something is!' and surprised myself that even then I could still find time for a laugh. I'm reassured. Now we just have to get the pain under control. A guardian angel called Rebecca arrives. She gives me Oramorph, tramadol, and a paracetamol drip and the pain drifts away like tides lapping back from the shore, it's the first respite I've had in eighteen hours. She tells me of her plans to be a GP and that she thinks it's vital to have a thorough understanding of women's health, especially things like endometriosis. She's with me for fifteen minutes and is able to see the woman in front of her, not a textbook. She asks questions, suggests a better combination of meds for flare-ups and wonders if I

might be more comfortable at home. On the journey back I think how lucky her patients will be and remember that most doctors are brilliant, you just have to find the right one.

THINGS I KNOW NOW

How to handle emergency endometriosis

• Pack a small bag – water, hot-water bottle, pain meds, snacks, phone charger.

• Don't go to hospital alone; it helps to have support and an advocate.

• If you are alone but need support you can request a nurse, chaperone or health assistant to be present while you have an exam (this may delay things but you should always feel OK about what's happening).

• The power balance is tipped way out of our favour when we're in this much pain and it's in this part of our body. We're often so desperate for it to stop we'll agree to almost anything and accept what they suggest. But if a doctor proceeds with something when you have said no or asked them to stop this is not OK.

• If you feel uncomfortable, anything is causing pain or you're worried at any point say something.

- Doctors are likely to follow protocol and this will involve an internal exam, where they take swabs and assess where the pain is. It may be necessary but you can ask them *why* they are doing it. What do they hope to find or rule out?

- If you would prefer to have a female doctor or someone more senior and specialist to do the physical exam you can ask (but it might mean waiting longer until one can attend).

- Ask your doctor: what should *I* do during a flare-up? Are cysts more likely with my type of disease? Do they recommend a particular hospital to go to? Are there any interim medications that would help while I'm waiting, or enable me to avoid going to hospital if the issue is not 'urgent'?

How do I work with this?

I have done many jobs while living with endometriosis: waiter, comedian, actor, writer, PA, typist, receptionist, driver. Some of these have been easier than others. The ones that required me to stand for a long time were more taxing when everything was swollen and sore and there were times when I nearly threw up into a vat of lamb tagine or leant on walls so as not to pass out. At office jobs I plastered temporary heat pads on my abdomen and dosed up on painkillers. On stage I used mind over matter and self-medicated with adrenaline and alcohol afterwards. None of these were great ways to manage it, but I have learnt a few things along the way.

THINGS I KNOW NOW

Tips for working with endometriosis

- **Keep hydrated**.

- **Have regular food/healthy snacks**.

- **Learn to say no to things sometimes**: surprisingly this may mean you can say yes to more long-term.

- **Heat helps**: if you're comfortable with people seeing heat pads or hot-water bottles at work then go for it, but if you prefer to be discreet get heat patches that stick on clothes or directly to your skin.

- **Keep moving**: sitting for a long time can exacerbate pain; get up as much as possible, even if it's just to get a drink and shake about.

- **Try not to have too much coffee**: I really need to learn this one, but caffeine can aggravate the pain.

- **Recognise when the day is too bad to go in**: try to see the difference between *really* having to and thinking you *ought* to keep going. One day's rest can help you recover quicker and get back to work faster.

- **Work from home**: this might not be possible but if you can, it helps preserve energy and you can be more productive on the days when you're feeling fragile but still able to work.

The kindness of women (age 15)

I'm on the television set of *The Royle Family*. My dad's friend Sue Johnston has somehow made it possible for me to do my work experience here and it is one of the most incredible two weeks of my life. It's my favourite show and working on it solidifies my love and admiration for Caroline Aherne and comedy. I always wanted to be a writer, but now I'm sure that comedy is what I want to do. Everyone is so kind and generous, and because I'm more mature than they expected (one of the perks of growing up fast) they've let me sit on set while they film and then go into the edit. It's amazing.

In week two my period comes. This is when I wish I'd paid attention to my cycle; sometimes not being prepared spoils the very thing you were desperate to do. But here it is, no point in being cross with myself as well. My head is swirly, my body unbalanced and I'm nauseous with the pain, but I'm determined not to go home. This is too wonderful to miss. I ask the medic if she can give me some paracetamol; she's sympathetic but she can't. The insurance doesn't cover medication for minors on set. The head of make-up, Christine, overhears us and quietly sneaks me some from her stash. She is an angel with cropped black hair. I could cry at her compassion. It takes the edge off, enough to finish the day, even if I vomit on the train home.

* * *

Ten years later I was at a dinner party hosted by my sketch-pal's mum, Jennifer, an evening for all the wonderful women she knows. There we sat, six young women at the beginning of our careers, at a table with these gods of comedy. I went up to the terrace where Jess (fellow Lady Gardener) was sitting with a blonde woman. 'This is Ele!' Jess exclaimed. She tells me this woman's dear friend has endometriosis and she hopes I don't mind but she's told her I have it too. We talk a little about what a rotten disease it can be. Then I ask her how she knows Jennifer; she says she's a make-up artist and works with her. 'That's funny,' I say, 'ages ago I met a make-up artist who saved me when I was in agony, before I even knew it *was* endometriosis. You might know her? Christine I think her name was.' 'That's me!' she replied. This woman was the black-haired angel from all those years ago, and this time I *did* cry. I leapt up and hugged her and told her how much she had helped me that day. It's not often you get to tell people such things but the universe can be odd and wonderful that way sometimes.

THINGS I KNOW NOW

- **Sometimes telling people can be great**: they can help and offer more support.

- **Confide in someone you trust**: it helps if someone understands, it reduces misunderstandings about your work ethic and they may also be able to cover for you or help you out if you have a flare-up during work hours.

- **Nothing is more important than your health**: I should have left certain jobs much earlier. They contributed to my stress and pain levels in a way I didn't fully understand for years.

- **You're allowed to STOP, rest and recoup**: don't feel guilty about this.

- **Work with stress**: it's impossible to avoid having a difficult boss or a frenetic work environment, but find ways to 'come down' from stressful situations. What coping strategies would help? Something nice to look forward to in the evening?

Writing with endometriosis (~~write~~ right now)

It's strange writing about something that's going on in your body while trying to ignore what's going on in your body so you can write. And it's even weirder doing it on copious prescription painkillers. These drugs used to have me dribbling in and out of consciousness, but rather shockingly I have developed some form of functionality on them. In fact I'm writing this on tramadol right now. I go from complete arrogance that what I have written might actually be decent, only for that feeling to vanish, like the puff of air in a glaucoma test. It is replaced with a nauseating sense that I have no business writing anything at all. My dad, a playwright and novelist, assures me that this isn't just the drugs – it's the writing process. But I'm not so sure. Anything that I have written before now (that was any good) wasn't done on tramadol and codeine. But if I don't take stuff I can't get anything done because the pain roars through me and even my eyes go blurry with it. The hardest side effect of the meds is the cotton-wool nature of my brain. I write too much and can't seem to edit it down. The words won't sit still, everything floats around so I can't quite grab it, and when I do it drifts away and I can't find it again. My mind is like a jumble sale; there is something good under it all but you have to have an eye for it and the patience to rake through. All the thoughts are muddled up and when I do find something I'm not quite sure that's what I came for. But if I keep turning up I might just get somewhere. I might even write a book . . .

The cost of it all

Financial worries can arise if you're having to miss a lot of work: if you're self-employed this literally means you're losing money, and if you're employed you may be at risk of having so much time off they either fire you or, if they're understanding, they'll let you take unpaid sick leave. Either way money becomes a huge concern and an underlying stress.

We rarely discuss the financial cost that comes with managing endometriosis and the anxiety it can cause. There are the usual costs that come with illness: prescriptions, hospital parking fees, private consultations for more opinions and like anyone when you're sick, you try a multitude of things to help make your life easier. But women with endometriosis often go to extraordinary lengths to feel better or at least a bit better than they do at that moment and for some the financial strains can be crippling. These costs include anything from specialist diets and vitamins to physical support like massage, physiotherapy and acupuncture and psychological support like counselling, hypnotherapy and meditation.

On the days when we can't stand up to cook we order takeout, which will probably make us feel worse but we need to eat. We take countless taxis from work or a party because of the pain and we just need to get home fast. We have to buy a whole new wardrobe because we've ballooned up or skinnied down thanks to the various medications. Then there are the expenses to keep ourselves sane: the Netflix and Amazon subscriptions, the audiobooks and online shopping. But these distractions come with a price. So do all the coffees we consume to get through the day, the things we buy to cheer ourselves up, the comfy shoes to replace all those beautiful heels you can't wear any more, the big knickers for the worst days, the skimpy knickers to remind ourselves we're still sexy sometimes.

And let's not forget the cost of trying to keep the endometriosis invisible: the make-up, the moisturisers for our dry skin, the laxatives and haemorrhoid creams when our bowels mess us about, the copious jars of Jolen bleach cream to counter the hormonal treatments. (Where did all this facial hair come from and why is it so *dark*? I can't see this side effect on the packet, Mr GP!)

You need money if you're ill

I am very lucky that I have supportive and generous friends and family, people who treat me to meals, lend me money, give me work, bring over nice things or comp me into their shows. During the times when I have been unable to work, it's been very stressful and upsetting, but I have had the luxury of having parents who were still working in good jobs, who could help me with bills, rent and medical costs (endometriosis is not recognised as a disability, so I couldn't claim benefits). But what happens to those who don't have this support?

What happens to all the women who don't have access to free and good medical care? Or those who can't get insurance to manage the condition because they have a condition to manage? Many medical insurance companies won't cover people with a pre-existing condition, and if they do, the excesses can be punishingly high. You need help but can't afford it and the very thing you need help for is the thing that is blocking your chances of getting it. It's a Kafkaesque system.

Even if you have insurance, many companies don't cover the type of surgery or medication some women really need, and it can be very difficult to get a policy that allows you to see an endometriosis specialist. In this situation women either have to find vast quantities of money to pay for it themselves or if they can't afford the right care they self-medicate with non-prescription drugs and struggle on without adequate medical support. I know women who have been in such pain and so desperate that they have taken way over the daily dose in one go just to get some relief. There will also be women across the world that don't have access to *any* medical support at all and somehow manage the symptoms alone.

It is not only barbaric to leave women in this state when there are things that can be done to manage the condition and live better with it, but also short-sighted to simply disregard women whose sickness reduces their capacity. Think what they could be achieving and offering to society if they were better supported?

What's worse is that the decisions about our complex systems, what medication and medical support is available, are often being made by people in political situations who still have archaic and misogynistic views about women's bodies and what they should and shouldn't do. In 2017 Lena Dunham wrote in the *New York Times* about the proposed legislation in the US that would allow insurers to deny access to birth control, something which many women rely on for endometriosis management:

For millions of women living with endometriosis, polycystic ovarian syndrome, cystic acne, migraines, uterine abnormalities and a history of ectopic pregnancies, birth control can be a crucial, even lifesaving, medical treatment. Hormonal contraception can control pain and bleeding by stopping or significantly shortening the length of a woman's period. It helps keep women with the disease happy, healthy and able to work.

Denying women access to such basic medication and help is discrimination against women because they are women. If there isn't a cure for endometriosis we should at least be doing everything we can to help women live with symptoms and limit the progression of the disease. Increasing awareness about things like endometriosis would help prevent or stop this stuff but if we don't speak up about it, no one will know it's even happening, and the injustices will continue to go on unchallenged. Disturbingly, women's reproductive rights are being increasingly challenged, limited and even reversed. It's vital that we remain diligent, push back and talk about this stuff. Women use birth control for multiple reasons, but the choices we make about our bodies should be ours, it's not for anyone else to decide.

Money and mental health

It's important to recognise that the financial costs that come with long-term illness can have an affect on your mental health and cause a lot of anxiety. You may become worried that you have more money going out than coming in, and what the consequences of this might be. If you are unable to work because of the symptoms, the loss of identity, routine and purpose can also lead to depression and despair and it's hard to see a way out. If you are relying on another form of income, such as support from family or a spouse, the lack of independence and autonomy can also have an effect on your self-esteem and having to be so frugal may mean you have to live a very limited life in addition to being unable to do stuff because you're sick, which can make you feel further isolated.

THINGS I KNOW NOW

- Getting into debt or worrying about money can exacerbate symptoms and affect sleep, work function, anxiety and mental health.

- Try not to ignore costs or bills. It's always less frightening to have knowledge and take control rather than ignore it and let them mount up.

- Do a budget, work out what you can afford and when.

- Talk about your feelings and concerns, ask friends and family for advice or speak to your medical team and ask if there is more they can offer.

- Share subscriptions with friends/partner for audiobooks, Netflix, etc.

- You don't have to try everything at once. Pick the best three symptom alleviators and try them first?

- Plan for flare ups; remember those lists I mentioned – they can really help reduce costs as preparing allows you to budget and avoid urgent, emergency spending.

18

Emotions and mental health

Endometriosis can have a huge impact on a person's emotional and mental well-being and this aspect is rarely given much attention. Perhaps this is partly due to a 'get on with it' attitude that has lingered from hardened beliefs around periods and women's pain but it could also be because it's hard to know what might help on an individual level, and what might be useful both short and long-term based on *your* experience.

Endometriosis can have a significant impact on your life and plans: major choices such as having or not having children, your relationships, your career, where you live, how you will finance medications or therapies. The quest for diagnosis or a suitable treatment alone can be very hard, but living with a condition that is sometimes unpredictable and fluctuating can cause depression, anxiety, low mood and low self-esteem. If you take strong opiates or hormonal treatments they can also compound these feelings and have an effect on your mental health. We can also feel despair if we're experiencing a prolonged flare-up, after an unsuccessful treatment or if we're missing out of lots of things because of the symptoms.

Recognising the emotional and psychological effects of living with this condition is really important, as these things can be managed and eased through therapy, coping strategies and other support. If we don't address the impact on our mental health it can also begin to aggravate the physical symptoms resulting in extreme fatigue, anxiety, insomnia and worse pain. For a long time, I felt there was no point in talking about this stuff because it wouldn't change anything, but over the years I have learnt that ignoring it or focusing on 'fixing' only the disease wasn't helping. I would have to learn to live alongside it somehow, and that included recognising the effects of endometriosis on my head and the rest of my body.

Endometriosis is stressing me out!

Stress causes elevated cortisol (the stress hormone) levels, which is part of the fight/flight response; your body perceives a 'threat' or potential danger so you have a heightened reaction to things around you. Cortisol is released from the adrenal glands, meaning you get a surge of energy to get through a situation. But if the body is managing one stressful thing (pain), it can't handle much more. So if there are stressful things happening on top of this, it's hard for your body to regulate because it's managing too many things. This might be why we get that whizzy feeling when it's all too much. Chronic stress can put an enormous pressure on your body and brain, which can make the pain and other symptoms worse. Other brain functions, like memory and learning, can also be affected, and it can increase your blood pressure and lower your immune function.

THINGS I KNOW NOW

We can't always avoid stress so . . .

- Be conscious of what might cause stress and try to plan around it.

- Find things that calm down your system: exercise, yoga, meditation, music, breathing techniques.

- Think about what help in the moment: take a few minutes away from the situation, walk around for a bit, listen to your favourite song.

- Try to get out and about; studies have shown that being around nature or being outside in the fresh air improves mental well-being.

- Try to make space for small joyful things during the stressful times: phone call with a friend, enjoyable food, something distracting?

- Make a list of priorities: firstly in order of what you think has to be done. This gives you some control over it. Then rewrite the list in order of what you really *want* to do and what would help you achieve this.

- Talk about it with someone who understands. Stress is always alleviated by giving it a voice – it lets out some of the

Frustration and despair. Often another perspective is useful and even if they can't offer advice, sympathy can be invaluable and lightens it all.

• Implement your strategies ahead of burning out and before *having* to lean on them as they won't work as well.

Are you lonesome tonight? (Today, all the time . . .)

Living with endometriosis can mean we spend a lot of time on our own, which also means it's hard to escape our thoughts and there's too much time to reflect on the past and ponder on the future. Pain itself is an isolating experience. *You* alone are the only one experiencing it and it's a strange feeling to be so *in* your body while also outside it; a sort of solitary confinement, with your own body as your prison.

If you're in pain for a number of days it can be very difficult to see an end point, but if you're also *physically* on your own for long periods of time it can make you feel very low and lonely.

THINGS I KNOW NOW

- Meditation helps stop the thoughts from churning round and round.

- If you feel spaced out find things to bring you into the 'present': draw, paint, ring someone.

- If you've been cooped up for a while or are taking strong painkillers, the world can feel overwhelming. When you *do* go outside - music, audiobooks, podcasts help with anxiety, especially in a busy city.

- Tell people you'd like some company; if they don't know you're feeling low they won't know to help.

- If you can't see people in person, find other ways to be with them. On the bad days I often FaceTime people who understand what's going on, so they will just talk to me (without judging how poorly I look or expecting me to talk too much).

Can't you talk about anything else?

It's not uncommon to become a bit self-obsessed if you've been feeling poorly for a while. It may feel impossible to talk about anything but the illness and its unjust consequences but the danger is if you get into this cycle it will also dominate the good times and make it hard for you to find any joy at all. It can become a vicious circle if you talk about it all the time, you can start to see it as the only thing in your life, which is depressing for you, but it's also difficult and not much fun for those around you. People may find it hard to know what to say or how to handle this, so they may avoid you or stop seeing you so much, which then reinforces the sense of isolation. This is not to say you *shouldn't* talk about it but try to remember you are not the disease and it is not the only thing you have in your life. While it may be having a big effect on you at this moment, it won't be like this forever.

You're not alone

Sometimes it's hard not to feel that you're on your own, that it's hopeless and won't ever end. I've felt that too on the worst days. When it gets this dark, try to remember it *will* pass. You have many people who love you and you will get through this.

I Thought I Was Alone But Now . . .

I imagine an army of women behind me.

Two hundred million sisters, friends, cousins, mothers, grandmothers and aunts.

They are silent but they stand behind me in solidarity.

They march with me into the appointments and operations.

They are calm and strong when I can't be.

They smile with encouragement and they will me on.

They know I can endure this, even when I don't.

If I turn around I won't see them for they are in my head and my heart.

But we're here together.

We will demand to be heard.

I imagine an army of women behind me, incredible and persistent.

I thought I was alone but now . . .

Frida (17–33)

'We can endure much more than we think we can . . . I am not sick. I am broken. But I am happy to be alive as long as I can paint.'

Frida Kahlo

A few weeks before I was diagnosed, my mum took me to see the film *Frida* and it changed me forever. Frida Kahlo was a Mexican artist and an inspiration for how to live (and boy, she lived) with 'chronic' pain. She suffered lifelong health problems: she had polio as a child and then at eighteen she was in a tram accident, which caused near-fatal injuries to her pelvis, back and upper body. Although she survived, she spent most of her life in enormous pain, enduring countless surgeries and her injuries meant she was unable to have children. She became reliant on painkillers and alcohol for relief and spent a great deal of time isolated, which influenced her paintings, many of which are self-portraits. While she didn't have endometriosis, her experience of pain and seclusion is familiar to me and her story reminds me that an amazing life can be lived despite all the misery. Frida's paintings are bright in colour, but their content is often anything but traditionally joyful; there is a personal pain, both physical and emotional in her work and they speak to me in a way no other paintings do. I have a visceral connection to them, particularly the ones about fertility, her body and suffering. She is able to transcend the agony and sadness to create something.

* * *

During the withdrawal of the anastrozole treatment I was very sick; barely leaving the house and unable to work. I spent an enormous amount of time alone. Although I already had coping strategies galore for the bad days, this was incessant and my usual distractions were becoming tiresome. What do you do when TV isn't enough? There are only so many *Law & Orders* you can watch before you start to feel crazy. I became restless and agitated and increasingly impatient with the endless days of achieving nothing. I was desperate to do something creative with the time, but I couldn't write in this fugue state, my head was too mushy. My friend Emma, a doctor, suggested I start painting again. I'd loved it at A level, but I hadn't done much since, there wasn't the time and it wasn't a hobby that combined easily with touring. I was initially sceptical of 'art therapy', but it felt like something I might be able to manage while I felt so ill. At first it seemed stupid and self-indulgent, nothing was any good, but something was urging me to continue. Then I began to do huge pictures, scratching and lashing the paint across the canvas and it became a way of getting something out, of expressing without words.

* * *

Painting has become an important coping strategy and distraction on the bad days; all that colour makes me feel brighter and creating something that wasn't here when I woke up gives me huge peace and helps with the restlessness. Painting is particularly useful as it can be done at your own pace, it means you produce something for your time but it's less exerting than other hobbies. It also helps me combat 'the fog' and distance that come with the pain and medications, and encourages me to stay in the present. It feels like I was born in the wrong era somehow; a fragile woman with creative tendencies locked in an unpredictable and sick body. But this lifestyle needs a fortune behind it: 'Alas sir, I am impecunious, but I need a patron and a maid to live with endometriosis!'

* * *

My favourite story of Frida is that of her determination to attend the first exhibition of her work in her hometown, despite being desperately ill. Her doctors instructed her not to leave her bed. So she got her friends to carry her in her bed to the gallery. How can you not be inspired by her mischievousness, defiance and desire to experience it all, regardless of the constraints of a body in pain? When things get really difficult or I'm overwhelmed by how much I'm missing, that this pain might break me, I think of Frida and remember what can be achieved in the face of adversity and I feel a bit stronger.

A bloody difficult woman

Have you ever been told you're being 'hysterical' or 'hormonal' when you're trying to express your feelings? It's a notion situated in deep misogyny; labelling women as over-sensitive or that we're over-reacting allows our experiences to be disregarded. As women we can internalise this perception so much that we daren't talk about the major things happening inside of us or how we feel, for fear we'll be accused of these things. So, if our emotions actually *are* affected by hormones then we certainly aren't going to talk about it, as it will just reinforce this idea it's 'hormonal' and not real, so we're more likely to be dismissed or mocked. But however much we try to repress these feelings it doesn't mean we don't still experience them.

I used to feel uncomfortable expressing anger partly because, as a society, we don't like angry women very much. Anger doesn't suit our traditional gender role, so we scorn women with terms like 'out of control', 'difficult' or 'a bitch'. But I also felt that anger didn't get you very far; being articulate or funny seemed to be better if you wanted to change things.

However, somewhere in the middle of writing this book, I started to get really angry for my younger self, for all the other women suffering, those missing school and work, those without adequate or any health care – that all this potential is being limited by this disease. I became incensed as I read about women who couldn't afford surgery, those who had been lied to and dismissed, those left to handle it on their own. I felt furious that there is still so much confusion and lack of understanding about endometriosis, that there has been so little progress in treatments and awareness since I was diagnosed all those years ago. Mostly I became enraged because it became clear that my experience could still happen very easily to another woman now and it shouldn't. It *should* be better by now.

Laughter is the Best Medicine But Anger is the Best Tonic.

And, man, am I angry that:

- I have to be quiet about it for fear of being told I'm 'hysterical' or because periods and pain are supposedly 'a woman's lot'.
- I get dismissed by doctors.
- I'm told to 'just get on with it' by people who know nothing.
- I'm made to feel crazy. I'm imagining it, fussing, expecting too much.
- I'm told wrong and contradictory information.
- I have to handle this level of pain.
- I'm told that the only options are invasive surgery or drugs that make me feel horrendous.
- I've been constantly encouraged to have babies *now* – regardless of whether it's feasible or the right time for me.

- I have to spend loads of money on things to make me feel just about normal.
- I have to be a patient patient.
- I have to say no and miss out on stuff.
- I'm offered quasi-cures by charlatans only out to get money.
- I'm wasting my life waiting in waiting rooms.
- That this pre-existing condition is mostly dismissed unless I'm trying get health or travel insurance – then they prick up their ears (and their bank accounts).
- I'm angry - I didn't used to be.

Don't look back in anger

Anger can be very useful for endometriosis. It can be a catalyst for change, give you purpose and fuel your quest for diagnosis or more tolerable treatments, but it's not good for your mental health to be angry long-term. This is not a shameful or 'wrong' emotion to have, but you need to find a way to express it or it will become destructive to you. However, suppressing or denying feelings doesn't mean they don't exist or that they will disappear. The tension caused by holding in stress, anger, sadness and disappointment will start to impact your body too and ignoring them won't work either after a while. Trying to put on a brave face all the time can become overwhelming and may lead to unpleasant outbursts or saying things you don't mean in frustration. It can also increase the pain, isolation and depression. So it's important to find ways to express how this disease is making you feel. Sometimes just acknowledging these feelings can give you some relief and control.

THINGS I KNOW NOW

- Write: a diary, or list your fears and feelings, or a letter to endometriosis; capture the madness and frustration of it all. It provides distance and can be cathartic.

- Exercise: a short walk, yoga, even just punching a pillow will help release tension and frustration.

- Joking or laughing about it diffuses tension, gives you perspective.

- Talk about how you're feeling to family and friends.

- If your emotions are all tangled up, perhaps you don't know where to start or just feel angry, sad or paralysed by it, you might need more support. Ask your doctor if counselling is available.

I'm missing everything

There may be times when there are harsh choices to be made about what you can and can't do and you sometimes have to be disciplined about our health. But it can be very disappointing if you're missing out on things a lot. There may be days when getting out of bed feels impossible and others where you buck up and pill-up and make it to whatever you've committed to, whether it's work or a wedding. But trying to plan your life around an unpredictable body can be exhausting and frustrating and it's difficult to handle the times when you have to cancel or miss out on things.

THINGS I KNOW NOW

- Try to remember that you're handling this better than you think. Could you get some more support, physically and mentally, to help you manage these complicated feelings?

- Is there anything that might give you comfort and make you feel temporarily calmer and ease the disappointment?

- Plan things to look forward to. It's hard not to be weary of the disappointment that comes with having to miss out on things, but try to look forward as much as possible. What *can* you do? Holidays, home visits during flare-ups, take-aways with friends, book tickets for something wonderful.

Make space for the joy

If you've been struggling with the symptoms of endometriosis for a long time it can sometimes feel like all you're doing is just about managing that and there isn't much pleasure or enjoyment going on. Trying to find joy can feel like *another* thing that *you* have to sort out when you're already struggling. I once went to a GP when I was really low, in high levels of prolonged pain, unable to work and feeling generally very overwhelmed. She told me to try and be more upbeat and suggested I read a book about how to find little joys in the everyday, concluding, 'I've really enjoyed it, especially with the weather being like this, it can get you down can't it?' I went for help and left with something for my Amazon wish list. But as infuriating and misguided as this was at the time, she wasn't completely wrong.

Endometriosis joy division

There's a lot of evidence that when you do something that makes you happy, hormones such as serotonin, endorphins and oxytocin are released and they can reduce pain signals and calm down your central nervous system. It may not always have a *physical* impact on the pain for you, but distraction and fun is hugely important for your mental health. Making space for the joy is a really important part of living with endometriosis.

THINGS I KNOW NOW

Over time it's easy to stop seeing opportunities for joy; invites to things, friends reaching out. Sometimes we can even perceive them as stressful or depressing because we fear we'll be disappointed if we can't do them because of a flare-up.

The trick is to think about what you *can* do and try to plan around the symptoms. Are there times when they're worse? Consider if the joyful thing might make a flare-up more likely afterwards, so could you do some and not all? E.g. you might not be able to go for the drinks after but you could go for the meal.

Discovering what coping strategies bring joy can take time, but here are some ideas of things you can do on your own or with others. They might seem small but sometimes it's the little joys that get you through on the more difficult days.

- **Listen to songs that remind you of nicer times**: turn the volume right up.
- **Watch/listen to/read something funny**: laughter is the best medicine remember.
- **Watch your favourites**: a film or box set snuggled up warm on the sofa.
- **Have a cuddle**: makes you feel safe and releases happy stuff.
- **Have a nice warm bath/shower/drink**.
- **Light a scented candle**: sounds daft but it helps with relaxation and decreases anxiety. Favourite smells also evoke happy memories.
- **Have a massage**: expensive treat but can be extremely therapeutic, especially after a flare-up. TIP: Some therapists run a co-op pricing scheme for people on lower incomes, or look into trainee/teaching sessions. Always mention the endometriosis so they don't aggravate anything.
- **Have sex/masturbate**: might be difficult at certain times of the month (or more often) but you can still have arousal without the potential pain of penetration. The oxytocin released makes you happy and relieves stress.
- **Ask a pal to do something**: things are always better together.
- **Go to the cinema**: go live in someone else's world for a bit.
- **Listen to the podcast you have been storing up**.
- **Do some online shopping**: if you can't afford it, just add it to your wish list for later, you get a similar feeling to buying.

I Dream

I dream
Of croissants and high heels,
Of dancing without the consequences,
Of trampolines and ice skating,
Of long walks and spinning around till I'm dizzy with the
    children I love.

I dream
Of lovers, and sex, and someone to hold my hand.
That I'm wearing all the clothes that sit tightly in a box under
    my bed – too small, too tight, too uncomfortable.

I dream
Of a stage and an audience laughing,
Of swimming out into the sea until I'm bored and wrinkled,
Of strength and joy and real exhaustion after a long day's
    work.

I dream
Of comfort,
Of being able to trust and rely on my body,
Of being carefree,
Of late nights and bad food and a one-day hangover.

I dream
Of waking up without pain,
Of never going to hospital again,
Of knowing what it's like to be young and normal.

I dream
Of never taking any more painkillers. Ever.
Of a different life to this one, the one I was going to have
   before it all began.

I dream
I'm a man, with none of this to deal with,
Of being a mother to children that only exist in my dreams.

I dream that this was a bad dream.
I dream, but I always have to wake up.

And way down we go (age 29)

They ask you about suicide a lot when you go to the doctor
and you have a long-term, painful condition. They say things
like, 'Have you put into practice any of your plans?' Which
immediately makes me think of a dress rehearsal. 'No,' I say,
'of course not.' This is somehow enough to reassure them,
like they just have to tick it off on a checklist. I haven't put
anything into *practice*, but I do have thoughts of ending it all
more often than I'd like, and that's not OK is it?

* * *

Last week the doctor offered antidepressants, but my body
feels like a mobile pharmacy already. I used to have scripts

rolling round my head and now all I can remember is the names of drugs and what time I can take some more. I don't think this is clinical depression; it's not a chemical imbalance in my brain but a perfectly natural response to every bit of my life being stopped. It feels like a sane reaction to an untenable situation. I can't work, I can't socialise, I can't go on dates, my career is disappearing faster than the swoosh of an email saying my body is too unpredictable to audition, even if it *is* for one of my favourite shows. The only theatre lights I'm under these days are when I'm in surgery. The misery can't be masked by more tablets. I asked if I could speak to a psychologist, but he told me the waiting list is over three months. 'Good job I'm not desperate,' I replied. Two days later I got a phone call to tell me my referral had been declined. I don't meet the criteria, I'm not sure why. She suggested I seek help privately, but I'm already struggling to pay for all the other doctors. My brain will just have to wait.

* * *

I've got all my painkillers laid out on the bed. I'm ashamed that I have been broken by such 'female' things as my uterus and my love for a boy, but I can't do this any more. I'm disconcertingly calm and rational. For a second I wonder if the drugs and hormones are exaggerating my reality, but I know this isn't something that will feel brighter tomorrow. I look at the pills again – I don't *really* want to do this. I call my mum; she talks me down. I go to bed with hiccups. In the morning I look up psychotherapists near me. Scrolling through I wonder if there might be someone who specialises in endometriosis. (I'm nothing if not still optimistic.) There isn't such a person of course, but I do see a woman with a kind face, and email to ask if she'll see me. A week later I sink down on a plush velvet sofa and tell her of my heart-ache, my uterus ache, my life ache. This woman saved my life.

* * *

There have been less lucid times when the pain was so bad I have thought it would be better to die than endure this for a moment longer but I had never felt I would rather end it all than carry on. The shock of getting this low jerked me into getting more help, but a different kind of help this time: not a body doctor but a mind doctor. I had been so absorbed trying to manage the physical effects that I'd suppressed all the feelings around it. It turns out that you can't view your body and mind as separate; they're talking to each other behind your back.

The endometriosis effect

There is still a stigma attached to therapy and seeking psychological support, as though it's indulgent or weak to ask for help. It's strange that we don't think twice about seeing a beautician for a wax, or a chiropractor for our bad back, but looking after our brains (and therefore our bodies) is different?

I have some amazing friends and family, and without them I wouldn't have got through any of it. But some of this stuff was heavy and my desire not to 'keep going on about it' had become overwhelming. I felt intense shame that I'd failed to resolve the situation, which was hard to acknowledge to myself, let alone to people I loved. Most of all, I couldn't bear to confess I had got this low, that I'd been unable to 'snap out of it'. Even with the best intentions there is also a limit to the support loved ones can give before they run out of advice and you might need the help of a professional. The impact of endometriosis on my life had become too difficult to manage on my own and I needed the skill of someone qualified to help me untangle it all.

I was lucky to find a therapist who was very good. She was kind, but most importantly she listened *and* talked, which was important for me. I didn't want to just rabbit on for an hour and leave; I wanted to discuss and work through it with someone. She helped me to see that while this was an impossible situation, I was handling it better than I thought and gradually I came out of the deep sadness I was stuck in. I hadn't realised how much I'd squashed down until it burst out of me: all the fear and anxiety, guilt, anger and disappointment, all the horrible doctors and bad news, all the pain and sadness, all that emotional and psychological trauma of living with this disease that I'd been holding in for so many years in order to keep going, to be strong, and not let it take over my life.

The first few sessions were exhausting and emotionally draining but slowly I began to feel slightly lighter, more in control. The anxiety and depression didn't just disappear, and I still get very low from time to time, especially when the symptoms flare up. But now I break it down into manageable chunks, focusing more on what I *can* do rather than what I *can't*.

I can also talk about this stuff more openly now (and even write a book!) and I'm better at asking for support without feeling I'm a burden. And guess what? The people who love me turn up; they give me a hug or bring cake and they try to help in some way, somehow. While the symptoms didn't change that much, I became slightly brighter each day and I slowly came to terms with actually living *with* endometriosis and all the trials and tribulations it brings.

Therapy has been enlightening and vital to my recovery, and I wish I had done it sooner. But my therapist would tell me off for telling you that, because it is a waste of energy to regret how you coped before, however dysfunctional your strategies were. I also know that when it comes to living with endometriosis you're only ready to try things when you're actually ready.

We need to talk about endometriosis.

- It's important for *everyone's* overall health to talk about feelings and fears, but with an inconsistent and change-able health condition it's vital to talk about how this is affecting you.

- Finding the right person and right type of therapy for you is key.

- If you're struggling but cannot afford private support, go back to your doctor and explain how much this is affecting you, that you *need* to speak to someone. In the meantime, there are services you can call if you're very low (see page 342).

- Your mental health directly affects the physical symptoms, both in a positive and negative way. This is something you can get help with, please don't suffer silently.

> • You are not weak. Living with a long-term condition that fluctuates, causes pain and has an impact on many parts of your life is hard to manage on your own. It is *normal* to ask for advice and help with this.

A sort of acceptance

I have had to adapt to the reality that endometriosis and pain will feature heavily in my life and it may present some limitations, but how I choose to *approach* this will determine how much it gets to affect me and my plans. Recognising this has been surprisingly therapeutic, not just mentally but physically, and it's given me more control over the symptoms. It's a constant juggling act to get it to a manageable place and I still push my body to do more than it wants sometimes, but I'm better at managing and listening to it. The disappointment when the bad days take over is not gone but I am more positive that they will pass now and have coping strategies to handle them more effectively. I am still baffled by my body's lack of stamina, but I have learnt ways to overcome this and join in still; I've got very good at shoulder dancing at weddings while I sit down and I can still laugh even on the hardest days.

While it's been difficult and distressing at times, there have been some very kind, clever and wonderful people dotted around in my journey too:

The doctor who squeezed my hand and said, 'I'm sorry you're going through this, but you'll be OK, I have a feeling.'

The pain psychologist who let me resist and rage then said, 'It's going to get easier, I think you might even write about it someday. I think you should.'

The specialist nurses who got me a sweet tea, listened and put their arm around me.

All the auxiliaries and porters who made me laugh.

The amazing women who share their stories and advice so I feel less alone.

The researchers who are passionate and told me they'll demand it gets better.

The friends and family that keep checking in and coming to see me when I can't see the light.

None of this fixes anything or changes the fact I have endometriosis, it doesn't always lessen the pain or make anything *actually* better but these moments of kindness give me strength to handle the next bit, whatever that is. Compassion costs nothing and we need more of it. Also hope, humour and joyous moments amongst it all are the only way to survive. So my best advice? Find ways to get these things into your life. This is how I really learnt to *live* with endometriosis.

Talking to myself

ME NOW: Remember earlier when I said you don't get given an endometriosis pamphlet?

ME 17: Yeah.

ME NOW: Well, it's a bit bigger than that but I think this is what you wanted, isn't it?

ME 17: Sort of . . .

ME NOW: Has it helped?

ME 17: Yeah. It's been a bit depressing at times though. I kind of wanted to know what it might be like but also just forget about it.

ME NOW: Tell me about it. Imagine trying to write the bloody thing!

ME 17: Do you have anything else to tell me that you might have forgotten? If not I'm going out dancing while I can.

ME NOW: You've not stopped dancing, but yes. Give me your hand . . .

ME 17: Why?

ME NOW: I want to squeeze it.

ME 17: OK, this is a bit weird . . .

ME NOW: You are strong, resilient and brave. You'll be able to endure the bad days and dance on the others. There is an army of women behind you, remember that on the days when it gets a bit difficult. I'm sorry you're going through this, but you'll be OK. I have a feeling.

Private Part(s):
the interviews

Lena Dunham

Interview: August 2018

Lena Dunham is an award-winning actor, writer, producer and director. Lena was diagnosed by laparoscopy age twenty-eight. In 2017 she had a hysterectomy to alleviate pain that wasn't being controlled by medication or more traditional surgery. In 2018, she had further surgery to remove her left ovary. I first spoke to her when I was very ill and she was incredibly kind (and of course made me laugh). It is an honour to include her here.

E: How long had you been suffering with symptoms before you managed to get a diagnosis and help?
L: My symptoms began at age twelve, two years before my period started – pelvic pain, cramping, intermittent crippling stomach aches. For the next sixteen years I experienced a baffling range of issues and a general experience of 'unwell-ness'. I just always felt 'off,' at first it was only when I had my period but, later on, it just

became constant. Good days are still the exception and not the norm for me. I try and focus on how lucky I feel about the magic in my life, but sometimes I'm really pissed and babyish and whiny about the realities of living with this illness. The only thing that comforts me is communicating with other endo gals.

E: Did you believe, like many of us, that painful periods were normal, so just tried to tolerate it, or did you keep pushing for answers?

L: My mother never had painful periods. My sister never had painful periods. My aunts and grandma seemed not to have painful periods. Yet still, I believed I was weak (or maybe because it was so easy for them, I believed I was weaker). It was hard to get anyone to really focus on the issue, but I was in too much pain to stop asking. By the time I was diagnosed I had seen at least five gynaecologists, a range of healers, gastroenterologists, therapists and masseuses. I would not wish the experience of having a 'medical intuitive' in Ohio talk in accents to your vagina on anyone.

E: How did you handle the symptoms during the undiagnosed years?

L: I did everything from copious Advil to hypnosis, drugs – legal and otherwise – ERs and days spent at home in pyjamas. It impacted everything from schoolwork to sex, mental health to what I wore. (For example, no jeans – I couldn't handle stiff fabrics. When jeans are too formal for you, you know you're in trouble.)

E: I know that feeling! Did you experience dismissal from doctors?

L: It's hard to get people to take a woman's pain seriously, even other women. When I was fourteen a friend told me periods aren't a reason to cancel plans. I figured she was either tougher than me, or her periods must have been a fuck of a lot easier, likely some combo of the two. In college I went to the school health clinic and tried to express just how bad my pelvic pain was, the resident nurse was sympathetic but her hands seemed tied. She suggested an IUD because it had helped her daughter with cramps, though she wasn't sure why. She said for some women, it made the cramps worse. She shrugged. Like, sorry, but that's not enough info for me, lady!

E: What's been the most successful treatment/combination of treatments for you over the years?
L: Honestly, it was a hysterectomy. I wish I had a better or more uplifting answer, but my uterus (which had essential structural issues beyond endo and really never stood a chance of doing its job) caused me more pain than I was able to bear. I became worn down and I basically related to my uterus like a bitchy childhood friend I couldn't shake. It was finally time to ghost her.

E: It's been vital for me to have a specialist doctor who listens and sees the person not just the disease. How long did it take for you to find your 'guy', and what made them good for you?
L: It took me eighteen years to find my guy, and that guy is Tamer Seckin, one of the world's premiere endo doctors. He's made a career out of listening to women. He's intense and creative and a real poet in how he thinks. I love how keyed up he gets about the injustice of how endo patients are dismissed and how aware he is of misogyny in medicine. We bicker.

E: What do you wish you'd known earlier about endometriosis?
L: I wish I'd known how different the illness is for everyone so that I didn't compare and wonder if I was normal. I would meet

other women with endo and think 'How is she so good at getting out of bed? Why am I such a weakling?' But no two endo cases are created equal and we get nowhere from judging ourselves – that's just more pain on top of the pain we're already in!

E: Are there any lifestyle changes you have made which help you to manage the symptoms?
L: I'm still figuring out what strategies actually improve my health but I will say that I never feel worse from sleeping more. Eating less sugar and caffeine helps. Getting massage helps. I have joint pain, so exercise can be tough but movement is good for keeping calm and keeping calm is good for pain and I've also noticed the more I love my work and my friends and my home the less pain I'm in because the mind–body connection is real as heck.

E: Have you found any alternative therapies helpful?
L: Acupuncture is a beautiful healing modality, and I also love the effects I get from Mayan abdominal massage. I'm sober and that's helped me focus on alternatives to medication because I try and avoid anything psychoactive (which many pain meds are), that's led me to seeing a naturopath and trying things like magnesium to relax muscles as opposed to Klonopin.

E: What coping strategies do you have for the bad days?
L: Sleeping is huge for me. Sometimes I need to just pretend I don't exist! And that's OK!

E: Do you take painkillers or do you try to avoid them and adopt a mind-over-matter approach?
L: I don't believe in trying to be a hero. Who does it help? Nobody ever went to heaven because they were so tough about their pain.

Who are we being tough for? I like to say 'I'm getting the epidural!' (Cuz if I could have a baby, that's what I would do.) Life is hard enough without adding false obstacles and denying yourself relief. Just stay honest with those around you about your relationship to medication and whether it ever feels like it's becoming problematic.

E: It can be a lonely condition, do you talk to friends and family about it? What is the best thing they do to help?
L: I never shut up. I talk and talk and talk. I wilt without talking – it's my oxygen, my water, my candy – it's how I survive. My father is an amazing listener and he always reminds me that this isn't fair, but also that it has made me more focused, humbled and empathetic (plus I am basically a gyno at this point).

E: Do you talk openly about it to colleagues or do you adopt an as-and-when-they-need-to-know approach?
L: I am probably too open. Like, maybe my male colleagues didn't need to hear all about the aftermath of having my cervix removed.

E: Were you always open about it or did you worry it might affect work opportunities or people's opinions of you?
L: I am not good at keeping my own secrets, I'm just not. So I really never felt I had another choice about whether to share this, or when. The inevitable conclusion was always to say it all, right away, much to my mother's chagrin. A few people have been dismissive. A few people have treated it as a professional liability. I'm very privileged to be able to say 'Thank u, next' (Ariana Grande-style) to those folks.

E: What advice would you give to men who love someone with endometriosis?

L: It's tough to remember that this condition isn't a reaction to you, sir, I know, but it's not. There's already enough trauma around sex with endo without you becoming convinced you're being rejected. There's already enough fear without being afraid you're going to leave us for someone who is 'able-vagina'd'. The loss of feminine identity that comes with this is as painful as the cramps. Please be gentle and please don't be squeamish (and buy us trashy magazines).

E: Have you had to adapt your life to accommodate this disease; your work, where you live, relationships?

L: Every damned day – I think about things most of my friends never will. A few examples: I can't travel anywhere that doesn't have good emergency rooms because I get cysts on my remaining ovary. I need to be able to plug a heating pad in at a work meetings without shame. My assistant usually double- and triple-checks that I know where I'm going and when I have to be there as pain can cloud my brain. The people around me need to know that when I cancel, it's not flakiness; it's beyond my control. Being in a creative industry is a wild blessing for me as an endo sufferer, but it can also be hard because the hours have zero regularity and I can't establish a healthy routine. A sixteen-hour day inevitably means sleeping for an extra eight hours the next. At this point, my health issues are super-public and that was painful at first because I felt like damaged goods but now nobody is shocked when I'm down for the count and that's helpful.

E: Pain and other symptoms, like 'the fog', can interfere with work, how do you manage this?

L: I try to be super-honest with myself and others about what I can do, and when I can do it. I'm an ambitious people-pleaser (weird combo!) so it can be tough, but I sure am pushing myself to really be clear every morning and night about how I'm feeling and what I need. I'm inspired by the brazen selfishness of old white men.

E: If you get a flare-up at work, so you're not able to rest, how do you handle it?

L: I just rest. I lay the fuck down. There's always an option, it may not be convenient for people, but without my health I'm useless. Again, I recognise the privilege of being able to demand a second to collect myself (or a week). I'm inevitably harder on myself than anyone else is and I'm learning to love myself like I'm my own mama.

E: I love that idea! Your work involves gruelling schedules and lots of adrenaline. Does it affect your symptoms? How do you get the balance right without 'burning out'?

L: I always feel on the edge of collapse but I also feel on the edge of creative nirvana. It's that dichotomy that keeps me going. I hope that as I get older and gain experience and wisdom I can work smarter rather than harder and tap into a little more wisdom about what makes me feel safe. I think that 'getting off' on stress and friction is very immature but I still see it in myself and it can take my pain from a 4 to a 10 in minutes flat if I don't watch myself. I wish I had a more inspiring answer!

E: Have you missed out on opportunities socially and/or professionally because of endometriosis? How do you handle the disappointment?

L: I have missed a lot – everything from hot dates with cool dudes to awards shows to fancy steak dinners and vacations and jobs. I try and focus on what a gift it is to be able to care for myself but I sulk, I cannot lie. I think my saving grace is that I'm essentially a homebody who thrives alone. I don't know what I'd do if I actually loved being social!

E: Has living with endometriosis changed your relationship with your body and have you found a way to live with it?
L: I have a real love-hate relationship with my body, always have. It is a very lonely thing to be human, to be trapped alone in corporeal form, and that's highlighted when your body is not kind to you. The only answer? Be kind to *it*, kill it with kindness, in fact. Don't punish it for what it can't do, love it for what it can.

E: It can have a big impact on confidence, and how we feel about our image, how do you handle that as an actor?
L: Endo has made me love to write even more than I already did. Writing lets me escape and be other people – in every way my body confines me, writing frees me. I'd probably love acting a lot more if I loved having a body. I think I'll act less and less as time goes on and I don't know to what extent that's a reaction to endo.

E: Some treatments have visible side effects, have you experienced this and how do you cope?
L: My weight fluctuates. My hair has fallen out. My stomach puffs. I get mega zits and puffy eyes. My sleep is interrupted. But I also have the kind of wild self-confidence that comes from knowing I am a tough, tough bitch who has lived through hell, and that makes me feel proud and valiant and stoked to be me. I think every woman, endo or no, is confused about who she is and how important her looks are to that equation. In a way endo is just a high-octane version of what we all deal with.

E: In your piece in *Vogue* (2017), you talked about having a hysterectomy and that it was not so much a 'choice' but the only way out of such pain. How are you feeling now?

L: I've had some great months and some tough ones in the year since my hysterectomy. Right now, today? I hurt – my scar tissue stings. I have back pain. My bladder is heavy. Yesterday was amazing though. I'm body bipolar but I am a strong believer in letting things take as long as they take. (Unless it's pizza. When I order pizza, it better show up fast.)

E: Your description of a 'choice' in a choice-less situation, strikes me as the epitome of the challenge women face with this disease, especially those with severe cases where drastic treatments are offered. Have you experienced the trial and error of multiple treatments?

L: I've tried so much. There have been countless 'solutions'. They're never the last solution. I've learned to expect progress not perfection, and I no longer frame things as 'the cure'.

E: Do you have any advice on how to handle the grief around infertility? I sometimes find myself choked up by incongruous reminders and it's overwhelmingly painful. Have you experienced this, and how do you handle it?

L: It's fucking hard and I never know when it will hit me. I have baby fever and wild jealousy. Starting to plan how I will be a mother is the only thing that's alleviated my pain around this. And I do believe I'll be a mom – and a super-fun, funny, cool one at that. Also, people can be such assholes about the infertility. I won't name names – you know who you are (or maybe you don't, LOL).

E: What advice would you give to a young woman who has just been diagnosed?

L: I would say: this is not the end of your life. In fact, it's the beginning because knowledge is power and you will soon be the most powerful witch of them all. Be kind to yourself and others. Be honest with yourself and others. Get a heating pad and figure out what makes you feel safe. Stay close to empathic people and get very comfortable saying the word 'uterus'. I love you!

* * *

Paulette Edwards

Interview: September 2018

Paulette Edwards is a BBC radio presenter and former English teacher of fifteen years. She was diagnosed age thirty-four. This is the first time she's spoken to anyone about living with endometriosis; I am flattered she chose to speak to me.

E: How long had you been suffering with symptoms before you were diagnosed and got help?

P. I had always had really bad periods, very heavy and painful from the age of ten. I was diagnosed when I was thirty-four, by accident when I had an MRI scan for another condition. I had cysts and one of my ovaries was so compromised that sadly I had to lose it. I didn't even know what endometriosis was; I'd never heard the word before if I am honest. I was shocked, surprised and a bit upset. But without that scan I don't think I would have known; the only pain I had was during my period.

E: Did you believe, like many of us, that painful periods were normal, so just tried to tolerate it, or did you keep pushing for answers?
P: I would have to have time off work and school. I'd feel sick or I'd pass out because the pain was so intense but I never went to my GP with it. I just thought that in my family it was normal because my mum always said she had really bad periods. As you know my family is Caribbean. My mum is Jamaican and she used to be a maid cleaning people's houses. That's how she made the money to come here. She remembers when she was cleaning people's floors crying with the pain. She used to sit on buckets of warm water to see if it would relieve the pain bless her heart, she was only fifteen.

E: Do you think your mum maybe had endometriosis too?
P: I don't know? It hadn't affected her fertility because she had six kids, but she did have a hysterectomy in her early forties. I am not quite sure why that was, I never really sat and talked to her about that. But that's what she suggested, she used to say, 'Why don't you sit on a bucket of water?'

E. Did you?
P. It was a pail; my mum always had pails because she did the terry-towelling nappies. She'd get some hot water in a pail and say, 'Just sit over that, it'll relax you.'

E: Did it help?
P: No! It didn't work and it was awful. Sometimes the water was too hot and you would burn there, it was horrible!

E: But your mum was understanding?

P: Yes, she kept me off school every month early on; she wanted to help me through it. But I think a bit of her felt, 'Well, I went through that and I was working and your life is so much easier. You will be absolutely fine!' I think I felt like I was a bit of a wuss, I couldn't quite cope with it. It's funny that barometer that we set ourselves for pain – if you can't handle this kind of pain, are you a woman? It's very sad isn't it? Because pain is pain. I know now that if you are experiencing period pains you need to go and see your doctor because that's not actually normal.

E: What coping strategies did you have for the bad days?

P: Staying in bed. Just sleeping, staying still. I tried clary sage once and I remember feeling so sick I vomited on myself in the bath. I couldn't control the pain, nothing I took touched the pain – ibuprofen, paracetamol – I would take so much I'd make myself sick and woozy but the pain was still there. I just thought I'd need to take more painkillers, which is terrible. It breaks my heart a bit for that young woman who was struggling through that.

E: How did you handle the symptoms while you were working as a teacher? All those hours standing up must have been hard?

P: I remember dreading my period and thinking, how is it going to work? Which day will I have to have off? Sometimes I would work through, but it was hard work and I had to manage my day. Having a room near a toilet helped – just for moments out. To be honest there were lots of tears when I was alone, I never seemed to have enough time for myself, pain can be exhausting. I tried to fight it because it seemed everybody else was all right. Sometimes I'd go to work and have to be taken home. I always felt really bad because I shouldn't have gone. It wasn't always easier because then you would have to explain to someone what was happening, I'd be a bit economical with the truth so they didn't feel embarrassed.

E: Do you talk openly about it to colleagues or do you adopt an as-and-when-they-need-to-know approach?
P: As-and-when approach. I wouldn't want to tell my boss that I have to stay in bed because my period is really heavy and I am in agony. One time I needed to go home my head teacher took me, he didn't ask me why. I think he had a bit of an inkling that it was 'women's troubles' – that phrase! [*Laughs*] More recently, if I have spoken about it in passing, a few people have recognised the symptoms through their experience and asked more questions.

E: Have you found any alternative therapies helpful?
P: Acupuncture has always helped to manage the pain. When I was nineteen, I did a meditation class about talking to and connecting with your body, it was quite weird. It takes you out of your body and right into your body at the same time – to find the bits that are tense. Because I think when you're in pain, you fight it, you tense so much it makes it worse. You have to do the meditation every day for a month and then when you have really intense pain you can use the techniques to almost 'switch off' the pain, it was the only thing that worked for me, it would just take the edge off.

E: Have you made any lifestyle changes that have helped your symptoms?
P: Exercise helped with the pain. I stopped eating wheat, which helped me to manage weight; I have found symptoms to be worse when I am heavier. I also gave up meat. I would say exercise had a significant effect because it made me feel better about myself, more positive.

E: Have you ever tried any hormonal treatments for endometriosis?
P: I took the pill for a year and I hated it. I always felt a bit invaded by the pill, my body didn't feel comfortable, didn't feel like it belonged to me.

E: So you were diagnosed with endometriosis accidentally?
P: Yes, I became ill with Benign Intracranial Hypertension; which is basically fluid on the brain, which was putting pressure on my eyes and sending me blind. So they fitted a shunt and did a scan to see if it was working. That's when they found that I'd got endometriosis. Then I had two surgeries, where they removed a cyst and whatever they do. It got rid of the ovulatory pain but not really the period pain.

E: Had the endometriosis had an impact on your fertility?
P: They said if you really want to get pregnant you'll need some assistance, which was scary, especially in a family where my mum says, 'I only had to look at your dad!' But neither the gynaecologist nor the neurosurgeon could tell me if IVF would compromise the other condition. They couldn't tell me anything that would make me think, 'All right, I will go ahead and do this.' I was terrified. The possibility of the other condition returning through IVF made the decision for me. I just thought I had had an awful four years with that condition and I didn't really want to go back there, I worried if I pushed it . . .

E: So you decided not to pursue fertility treatment?
P: If we'd got pregnant naturally I would have been ecstatic, but to force my body, I didn't feel was for me. Sometimes I think I didn't make the right decision but mostly I think it was right for me at the time.

E: How have you coped with the effect on your fertility?

P: It does affect your mental health; it makes you feel less. Sometimes I don't even talk or think about it because it's a bit too painful. I go through phases. I went through a nappy phase, where every single time there was an advert with a baby on I would cry, every single time. And you know what my partner did? And this is a bit weird but I love him for doing this, he bought me a doll. Because there are times when I want to, I don't know what it is really, I don't even know if it is good for me but sometimes just having a baby-like figure in your arms kind of just takes the edge off it a little bit, it helps with that sense of loss, that grief in a way It doesn't stop me crying, I cry all the time. If I see a newborn, I cry. When friends have babies I dream about them, it wakes the feelings up every time. It's as if you are grieving for something that you never had. I'm maternal, I feel like I'm a mum but I haven't got children.

E: It can be hard to share some of this stuff, do you talk to friends and family about it? What is the best thing they do to help?

P: The infertility was hard to talk to my mum about, she never had any trouble conceiving, so there was a lot of pressure from her about having children. I have some great people in my life, friends and family, but I have never had this conversation with any of them, I have never been this honest about my fertility. I am probably talking about this for the first time like this because my friends are at different stages, there are a few who haven't had children, and we can't even talk about it because it's too raw.

Interestingly now I'm more open about why I haven't had children, women who have issues with fertility will come and have a chat with me. I am always happy to do that because I would have been grateful to have spoken to other women with the condition. I didn't really understand what was happening.

I have had friends, usually ones who don't know me very well, who haven't been very thoughtful. But those that know me very well, I have always been part of their children's lives. I really like that. They are very sensitive without asking much. The friends who know me want me to be a part of it all but those who don't know me as well won't even tell me they're pregnant and that upsets me, not so much now but it used to really upset me.

E. Because you're sort of being excluded twice?
P: Yes. You're very good at articulating things.

E. I've had to get good – I'm writing a book! Has living with endometriosis changed your relationship with your body?
P: My other condition made me grateful for my vision and my mobility, I was just grateful that I survived. But I felt let down by my body, endometriosis felt almost like a punishment, it's a horrible thing to say about your body, I don't really mean it, but that's how I felt at the time. I'd talk to my body sometimes saying, 'What's wrong with you? What have I done to you? There are times when I feel profoundly sad about not having children but usually I accept it.

E: Have you missed out on opportunities socially and/or professionally because of endometriosis?
P: I don't think I have but I have pushed myself harder than I should have and felt guilty about taking time off for appointments and surgery. The disappointment over fertility has been a harder sting to recover from . . . I'm mostly OK with that now.

E: Have you had to adapt your life to accommodate this disease: your work, where you live, relationships?

P: Maybe relationships. I was relieved to meet someone who already had children and supported whatever decision about whether to pursue IVF. I was always careful about challenging myself too hard in case I couldn't meet a goal I'd set myself.

E: What advice would you give to a young woman who has just been diagnosed?

P: Try to make choices based on how you feel and know *your* body. Be kind to yourself in whatever way you can. It can be hard when you're in pain and feeling vulnerable but ask questions from the professionals. Talk to others who have it if you can, everyone's experience is different, but sharing stories is really powerful and there will be something in there that will resonate with you. Some people find support groups helpful and others think they're a waste of time. I don't think they're useful for everyone. You need to be doing what's OK for you.

E: What do you wish you'd known earlier about endometriosis?

P: I had never heard about it before, I bought one book and I didn't read it. It would have been great to speak to someone else who had the symptoms. I wish I'd found out more about it, how massively it would affect my fertility and how to manage the pain. I wish I'd talked about it more.

* * *

Hilary Mantel

Interview: July 2018

Dame Hilary Mantel is an award-winning author and playwright. She once said that, 'Anything I have achieved has been in the teeth of this disease.' She was diagnosed aged twenty-seven. I first met her when I was at my lowest, her kindness has helped me get to where I am today, and she has become a generous friend since. To be able to include her story, wisdom and insight here is a great joy.

E: How long had you been suffering with symptoms before you were given a diagnosis and help?
H: I think the condition was there when I had my first period at eleven. I had a great deal of pain during my teenage years but I didn't complain of it. That's a cultural thing – you didn't. I was told it was normal for women to suffer in this way, and I didn't approach a doctor about it. I could not imagine approaching our family doctor. I blamed myself for not being tough enough. I didn't actually get a diagnosis until I had surgery at the age of twenty-seven.

E: So you handled the symptoms for all those years without support?
H: When I was eighteen I went on the contraceptive pill. After a smear test, my GP thought something was wrong and referred me to a gynaecologist. He was avuncular and kind, reassuring me that I didn't have cancer. But I remember very clearly what he said: 'If

you want contraception, the best thing for you is the pill.' I now realise he probably knew I had endometriosis, and I believe that is why he impressed on me to stay on the pill.

E: But he didn't tell you he suspected this?
H: It seems he didn't think I needed to know. It took me years to fit this together. The GP had seen endometriosis or more likely something she didn't understand. The gynaecologist thought (as people did) that being on the pill would contain or cure it. Looking back, I see this as the essence of patriarchal medicine – well meaning, but disastrous. It was as if he thought, 'No point in scaring this little girl.' What he should have said is, 'Stay on the pill – and here's why.' I saw another GP at the age of nineteen; I wasn't complaining of period pains because I was on the pill and the pains were mild. What I was complaining of was pain in my legs, nausea, fatigue, a general state of feeling I was ill in some unspecific way. But of course it was the endometriosis. There was no physical investigation. I was given drugs to address my psychological state. Antidepressants and medication against anxiety. Stupidly, I took them.

E: Had you come to think this was psychological then?
H: All my life I have been described as over-sensitive, so I thought it was my personality that was at fault. The story I was being sold was that what was happening to me was normal, but I was inter- preting it as illness. So it seemed that what had to be addressed was psychological rather than physical, which was of course a huge mistake, and led to the waste of many years. After that I didn't really want to go to a doctor, because of course no one likes to be dismissed in that way. However, I did go – back and back and back, as I got worse. But once it's written in records that you have been prescribed drugs to address a psychological condition, no busy GP

pulls back and asks, 'Could this be a physical illness, after all?' It was simply a matter of reaching for the prescription pad as before. I wasn't against drugs. I would have taken anything that would have helped me. The experience of those years wrecked my university career – intermittently trying to cope with the side effects of the drugs, plus the primary problem, which no one could see. I came to a point where I would not take any more drugs to medicate my state of mind. I wish I had come to that point sooner. When I look back to nineteen, twenty, it's just a horrible blur. I think, 'Why didn't you assert yourself?' But that is easy to say, looking back now. At the time, the more I said I was ill, the more it was treated as a symptom of my anxiety.

E: So the pill provided some relief?
H: Yes, but when I was twenty-four I stopped taking it, because I realised that my condition must in some way be hormonally controlled, and I wondered if it was the pill itself that was the problem – causing nausea, and so on. It seemed a worthwhile experiment to stop. Immediately, from the time my natural cycle recommenced, the pain got much, much worse. But I didn't know what to make of that. There was no one to help or guide me. In those years there were continual scare stories about the pill, and no one thought they could stay on it for life. I wonder now: was this science speaking, or culture? That women should have so much control over what had been seen as 'biological destiny' caused deep disturbance. I know now that moral judgements are often disguised as medical ones.

E: Had anyone ever suggested endometriosis to you at any time?
H: When I had come off the pill, and a painful cycle had re-established, it became clear to me for the first time that this was a gynaecological problem, despite the variety of symptoms. When

I was twenty-five, living abroad, I told a new GP about my monthly pain. Very sympathetically he said, 'You shouldn't be suffering like this.' This was the first time any doctor had believed I had a physical problem and expressed a wish to help me. I was immensely grateful when he gave me anti-spasmodics, which helped a lot. But of course they did not address the cause. I was so relieved to be listened to, to have someone take me seriously, that I didn't push further. Again, that was a mistake. This was the late 1970s. I hadn't even heard of endometriosis. The treatment masked the condition for another couple of years, until the pain grew over the top of what the GP prescribed.

E: So your symptoms were no longer cyclical, you were suffering daily by then?
H: Yes, that was the problem. The medication worked, but behind that masking, the condition was running on. Again, as when I was a student, it was manifesting itself in pains in my back and legs, constant fatigue and nausea. But these things, they are such generalised complaints, you can't honestly expect a GP to do much with them. And in those days endometriosis did not come to mind as a cause.

E: So how did you work out that this was a condition, that this was endometriosis?
H: It was not until I decided to pursue my own research that I heard of it. I was living in Botswana at that time. In the university library in the capital I found a textbook which graphically illustrated a female body in pain – a body with endometriosis – with lines like long pins pointing to the common sites of disease. It all began to add up. I think there was one textbook on endometriosis in those days. There was nothing written for the layperson. But I knew enough to understand that this was probably my condition.

E: Did you think 'Yes, that's it! That's what I have'?

H: Yes, yes I did! I also recognised that a lot of my psychological distress over the years had hit me the week before my period started and that there was a pattern of hormonal activity that accounted for so much in my life. I also had premenstrual migraines, but I'd never kept a diary, so I didn't see the pattern. But suddenly everything began to fit together.

E: Did you rip out the page and take it to the doctor, demanding they listen now?

H: There was a problem in those days – informed patients were not generally welcomed, and intelligent women had trouble navigating the medical system. Doctors were keen to tell you, 'Yes, you may be intelligent, but you are not intelligent in *my* sphere. Here, I am the boss, I am in charge of your body.' I do feel that was the case in those days, you were expected to hand over your body and your being to an expert – as if the expert wasn't *you*. There has been a cultural shift among doctors since that time, but that shift is still in process, and sadly it doesn't seem to have speeded up the diagnosis of endometriosis very much.

E: But it must have been a relief to finally know what was causing your symptoms, to have a name for it, that it was *real* and presumably there must now be a 'fix'?

H: Not really a relief, because I was still the only one who knew. So now I was going to have to think what to do, and that wasn't simple. I was bleeding all the time, which strangely was helpful, something is demonstrably wrong, there is objective evidence, and a doctor has somewhere to start. As I said, I had been working in Botswana with my husband, but we were due for leave, so we came back to the UK and I went to see a gynaecologist privately in

Manchester. He accepted that I had endometriosis and thought I needed to have an ovary removed. I remember him saying, 'If you are resident in Stockport it will be six months before you get the procedure. If you are over the border in Manchester, it will be never.' I think in that case I would soon have turned up in A&E as a surgical emergency, because, as I was soon to realise, I was in a very bad state, and could have developed peritonitis. Luckily, I was able to have surgery in London. I was advised to go to St George's Hospital, where they saw me when the pain was at its worst, and so took me in over the Christmas period. Looking back I recognise I was at crisis point, but when you are accustomed to crises of pain, you think of riding each one out. You don't think, 'Where is this going?' You are just so relieved when you get to the other side of it. You think in a superstitious way that maybe it will never happen again.

E: Yes that's it, you think 'I've done it now, I won't ever have to go through it more than this—'
H: Yes, you think 'I survived that!'

E: And it can't possibly get as bad as that again. I think that's a psychological thing to protect you from the memory of the pain.
H: Also, I think it is something to do with the nature of abdominal pain, pain deep in the body. You can't actually see it happening, and either you have got it or you haven't – and when you haven't, you are a different person, you're living in a different world.

E: So the doctors at St George's believed it was endometriosis?
H: I had scans for the first time, which revealed abdominal masses, they decided it was serious, but they didn't know what it was. They told my husband it might be cancer. So I went to surgery with no one knowing actually what was wrong, but in theatre it was obvious

that endometriosis was the problem. When I woke up I was minus both my ovaries, fallopian tubes, womb, a bit of bowel, a bit of bladder. But obviously, I had given my consent for them to do what they thought best. I am not complaining about that.

E: Had they told you this was a likely outcome?
H: I had an inkling, but only because the temporary GP I was seeing at that time – a very wise man who I wish I had met earlier in my life – said, 'I think they will remove your womb as well as an ovary if they find it's really bad.' I just could not compute that – a hysterectomy, that was a word I associated with women of my mother's generation. So because this good man warned me, I didn't have a shock, but at the same time I did not know the implications of losing both ovaries at twenty-seven. I don't think anyone really addressed the matter. The only time they talked to me was when I was still recovering from anaesthetic. They considered, and I of course considered, that whatever my new situation, at least the endometriosis was gone. This was not true.

E: Although the documents we sign before surgery warn that hysterectomy is a possible risk, it is impossible to know what you'll feel like if it happens. How did you cope with this when you woke up?
H: The documents I signed were a general consent. No doctor had felt able to specify what they might do, because they didn't know the nature of the problem till the surgery was underway. Afterwards I felt a strange sort of relief, I could point to the ultrasound scan and prove that those years of pain were not imagined. I felt this powerful sense of vindication and the possibility of a fresh start. I was stepping into the unknown, but I wasn't pessimistic. I had no reason to be. People were representing to me that 'This might

be drastic, but it had to be done.' Nobody suggested there could have been an alternative. I'm not holding anything against the surgeons. I think it is just the fact that we were all in a condition of ignorance.

E: Did you ever seek support from other women living with it?
H: About three years after the surgery, I realised the condition had come back. We had moved on to work in Saudi Arabia, and quite coincidentally, at a neighbour's house, I picked up an old copy of *Good Housekeeping* and there was a mention of a self-help group that had been formed for endometriosis sufferers. I immediately got in touch. This group later became the National Endometriosis Society and then Endometriosis UK. But until I met these founder members, that little group of women who set the whole thing going, I hadn't met anyone else with the condition. Meeting them was hugely important, because they had information, and it confirmed what I believed; that yes, it could come back.

E. Had the doctors told you that it *couldn't* come back?
H: They hadn't told me in so many words, but I had been led to believe that once your ovaries were removed, that would finish it off. I had been given oestrogen replacement, to prevent later problems with osteoporosis. It became obvious that in that first operation the doctors had removed what they could see, but that wasn't the whole of it. I don't mean they did a bad job, but the condition exists at a microscopic level. They were looking at the obvious places, the common sites. But there are other sites, less obvious, that may have been affected. When I was twenty-nine–thirty, I saw a gynaecologist in London, who was very reluctant to admit that the condition could come back. She blamed the pain on my bad marriage! [*Both laugh*]

E. So again psychological?

H: Well yes, and she made quite peculiar assumptions about my personal life. But she began drug treatment, she put me on a drug called Provera, which had the most dire effect on me. I took it for nine months, during which time my weight increased by about 50 per cent. I was 7 stone 3 pounds when treatment started. I was 12 stone-odd by the time she accepted I should be taken off it, and it had done nothing for me at all. The next month the condition was back as bad as ever.

E. It's hard to deal with when the drugs make the endometriosis visible, how did you cope with that?

H. My experience of drug treatments was like yours, in that it was obviously completely the wrong thing for my condition, and when my doctor understood the effect it was having on my whole body, she should have just said 'stop'. But I feel it was a matter of pride with her, she didn't want to be wrong. She herself was massively overweight and she also said, when I mentioned weight gain, 'Now you know what it's like for the rest of us.' Then she put me on danazol, which was then a new drug. There were very nasty side effects.

E. How long did you endure them for?

H. I had a stroke of luck, and I was due one. I saw a GP in Jeddah and it turned out that he had worked on the trials of danazol, he said I was on far too high a dose. He could tell just by looking at me. My whole body was swollen – I am not talking about fat, I am talking about oedema.

E: So did a lower dose help at all?

H. Drastic though the treatment was, I think it damped down the condition, and my worse days in some respects were then behind me with endometriosis *itself.* But then I began to suffer from the cure, so to speak – the fact that I had lost my ovaries. Thyroid failure is now recognised as more frequent in women who have lost their ovaries than in the general population, but when my thyroid failed I found it very difficult to get a diagnosis, because lab tests showed my levels were at the lower end of normal. Only later did I find out that the scale is very wide – it might have been normal for somebody, but it wasn't normal for me. I had to go and see an endocrinologist privately before I could get treatment. I was in a situation of incredible frustration. It was so obvious simply from looking at me that I had a thyroid deficiency. But of course in those years doctors had stopped looking. They just looked at their screens or down at their desk. I had the textbook signs and symptoms, but the evidence of the lab tests was privileged over the evidence offered by the patient's body.

E: Were you able to work during this time?
H: Until the thyroid deficiency was corrected, I was struggling to work. What made me desperate was the effect on my brain function. I was working longer and longer hours, and going round in loops. I remember writing an article that I meant to be about five thousand words, which came in at fifteen thousand words because I couldn't make it shorter. And all this flowed from the original condition. It seemed the drugs I had been given against endometriosis had messed up my metabolism in some way I have never been able to fathom. And no one has ever helped me to understand it. Also I got renewed crises of pain, and in 2010 I had abdominal surgery, which uncovered a huge mass of adhesions. It seemed that the endometriosis must have continued for many years. That surgery was complicated, and it took a couple of years for me to get over it. But then I had a better spell, better than I had ever been in my

adult life. But perhaps that's not saying much. My general health is fragile. It seems to me everything has followed in a long string of complication, from my teenage years when I failed to get a diagnosis.

E: You have talked about being unable to do a 'normal' job with this disease. Was the decision to make writing a career in part because you can work around the symptoms, have more flexible hours and work from home?

H: Yes. It was a choice to commit to it, to say not just 'I am going to write' but 'I am going to write *this* book'. I think it was a distinct commitment, and I made it at the age of twenty-two. I had hoped to be a lawyer, but I recognised by the time I left university that I wasn't strong enough for many careers. When we went abroad, then writing was a portable career for me. But of course it was a long time before I published anything. I was writing for twelve years before I made any kind of breakthrough. Sometimes people say to me, 'You wouldn't have become a writer if you hadn't been ill.' But it is complete nonsense to talk as if the illness somehow fed one's writing, all it does is obstruct and get in the way, make my life incredibly difficult, and there is nothing positive about it at all. However, with effort you can make a space in your life where the illness doesn't dominate everything.

E: Is there comfort in escaping into another world? Does it help you to transcend what's happening in your own body in some way?

H: No, I don't find anything comforting about writing. [*Laughing*] No, I find it extremely hard work! But it has allowed me a measure of power and control. I do take satisfaction in the fact that despite everything, I have been able to build a career.

E: Pain and other symptoms, like 'the fog', can interfere with work, how do you manage this?

H: The nature of bad days has changed, because I am not now routinely in pain, but what I have had to come to terms with is my general debility, weakness and the problems caused by weight gain. With difficulty and hesitation, I have begun to learn when to battle against fatigue and when to rest. My problem now relates not so much to the daily battle to get the words on the page, but to my public persona. I get wonderful invitations to travel, for instance, but I have to accept the restrictions on myself. There is a problem for endometriosis sufferers, in that it's not a visible condition. You don't look as if anything is wrong. You can hardly say to people, 'I can't do that, I don't have very good health,' without going into explanations. I must say that, that problem has dogged me throughout my career.

E: So you didn't confide in colleagues that you were suffering?

H: I remember very well when my agent rang me with a wonderful travel proposition and I thought, 'Now I've just got to tell him.' I talked to him for an hour. It never needed to be mentioned again. That was about ten years into my career. Before that I just toughed it out really, and I responded to things case by case. I did and continue to do things that cause immense strain, though I know that the best way to live is quietly. But you can't always stay at home.

E: Has this condition affected your relationship with your body?

H: I always feel that my body is unreliable. I have had just enough good days – days when I wake up and nothing is wrong at all – to know how 'fine' feels. It is like the sweet apple on top of the tree, it's like the crystal mountain, it is like a vision of ecstasy. There is normal, average everyday good health – and most of the time I am shut out of it. I think it is almost all traceable to endometriosis.

E: Have you found any alternative therapies helpful?
H: Many years ago I took an eight-week course in a relaxation therapy called autogenic training, which proved a very good investment of time and money (but don't try to learn it from a book). I never felt the pain relief I was given was very effective, and of course opioid medication has undesirable side effects of its own. The autogenic therapy helped me cope without routine analgesics. I don't practise the exercises every day, but they are a resource for me. I think what was important was that at that point, the mid-1980s, I was taking charge of my condition. I was not looking to the doctor for help; I was helping myself. I have noticed this from what other women have told me, there is a point when you take charge. Perhaps the particular therapy you choose is less important than the fact that you are actively seeking solutions outside the orthodox treatments.

E: So you'd recommend looking into alternative ways to manage symptoms?
H: I heartily recommend that people investigate complementary therapies. If what you need is surgery, they won't take away the need for that. But they can help you manage symptoms, or live with the side effects of drugs, and from day to day even temporary and partial relief is worth a lot. You need to boost what's positive in your life – anything that reconnects you with your body in a way that is not pain. You have to understand that it is worth giving yourself that attention, that time, that money.

E: With regards to endometriosis and fertility, I wonder if you can give some advice on how to handle the thoughtless things people say like 'Oh well, you can adopt'?

H: Sort them out! [*Both laugh*]

It can be difficult when you feel it is well meant, but you know, often it isn't. They can be sneaky, insidious questions, and the more successful and OK you appear, the more people are inclined to insinuate, 'Ah, but there is something missing in your life, isn't there?' In my time, certainly, I have tried to do the tactful thing, by backing out of the conversation rather than engaging with that person, but if I had my time over again I would engage. I would put them straight and stop them in their tracks, so they don't do it to another woman. It's easier for me now, because I have got to that stage in my life where I don't care what anyone thinks. I've stopped trying to be liked; I have entered my Germaine Greer stage! [*Both laugh*]

People are frantic to know why you don't have children. I think the hardest time for me was in my thirties, when I was living abroad, surrounded by women who were full-time mothers; necessarily, as in Saudi Arabia they had little chance to be anything else. I remember saying to a friend at home, 'I am so tired of being asked, "When are you going to start your family?"' She said, 'When you get back to England and you move into a different set of people, it will not be a question they ask all the time. They will know you as a professional woman.' And I found that that was true.

I don't know what the answer in your case will be, because I don't know if you are someone who would really like to have a child? But in that case you say to people, 'Well yes, I would like to have a child, but I am unable, because I have a condition called . . .' It's an educational opportunity. If you feel strong enough that day to take it.

333

E: I find talking about it hard because it's painful but also it's awkward to talk openly about a condition that affects such private parts of my life, especially with a stranger at a public event like a wedding.

H: At weddings, yes! That's interesting it's at weddings. Remember the power of the monosyllable. 'Do you have children?' 'No.' 'Are you going to have children?' 'No.' Shut it down. But if people say 'Have you thought of adoption?' they deserve all they get.

E: Hmm I am starting to feel that.

[Both laugh]

H: Hooray! Looking back I wish I had been tougher. But as you say, it's a matter of context. Where somebody brings it up at a wedding, you don't want to bring proceedings to a halt by giving them a lecture. But you can always find a way to make a point. For me it wasn't ever a question of being able to say to people, 'I haven't got children yet,' because I knew I was never going to have children. I wasn't on the fertility trail. I never went through that, I was spared all that. When people talk to me about this condition, often they know that I have no children and it's because of medical issues, but they assume that I've either had a lot of miscarriages, or I've been through fertility treatment, but no, actually this isn't me at all. There has been an assumption that if you haven't got a child, then you must be in pursuit of one – this must be your story. For me, the thing was it was done and dusted in one morning. I was a woman who thought she could have a child, but when I got out of the anaesthetic I was a woman who never would.

E: I can't imagine what that loss felt like when you woke up, how did you come to terms with this?

H: At the time it was the incapacity that upset me – it wasn't so much feeling the loss of a child, it was feeling the loss of possibility. It's that certain paths were now sealed. I think that is quite hard to come to terms with at twenty-seven. But my story is very untypical in that way, because normally the loss creeps up on people gradually.

E: Does the feeling of loss ever abate?
H: You feel it differently at different ages. I lack the markers of other women's lives.

The markers are not just the births of children, but that they go to school, they leave school, go to university, get married and then . . . then a new phase begins. One thing people say, 'Haven't you done enough now? What else is it you want? Why are you still so ambitious?' They don't put it quite in those terms.

E: That not having children means you overcompensate or are more ambitious? As if your work is instead of having children?
H: That's another question that I had to confront when I was younger, and I still get interviewers who go, 'You haven't got children, but you have got your books!' No one would ever suggest to a man that his career was undertaken to make up for lack of children.

E: Paradoxically you have felt *better* as you have got older?
H: The surgery in 2010 made a big difference. Three years on I was the best I've been, and it opened up opportunities to do things I'd wanted to do, like working in the theatre, that I couldn't do before. I found I was able to work the same hours as other people – not without strain, but I could do it. But at the same time I know that I still have to evaluate the possibilities every day. Like many people with long-term illness I have to do a mental scan of myself

335

and calculate: what can I achieve, and what am I likely to suffer? Wouldn't it be a blessing sometimes not to think about your body? [*Both laugh*]

E: What's the best advice you could give somebody who has endometriosis?
H: Get the best information you can. Put yourself on a footing of equality with your doctors. Know that if you really do your home-work you are likely to be better informed than they are. You don't have to take up a belligerent stance, but you have to take up an equal one, and keep on questioning, keep asking for second opinions. All that's fairly obvious. What I would say, out of my life experience, is try not to hate yourself. Just regard yourself as a woman who is doing her best, and anything you can do to keep your morale high, go for it. It's not self-indulgent, it's absolutely necessary if you are to live your life successfully, as I think you can.

Of course, that advice is absolutely no good at all to people who are in the throes of a bad attack, or sitting in A&E.

But in the long-term I want to say to people – you are still worth-while. When you are suffering and have suffered for a long time it's very easy to regard your body as trash, or as an alien working against you. Often women with endometriosis, especially those who are infertile because of the condition, represent failure to the medical profession. Pain also represents a challenge doctors cannot always meet. Naturally, they turn away from what they can't help. But you have to remember to assert the fact that you *are* worthwhile and *as* entitled as any other patient. You may be a failure to your doctors, but you can still set your own terms for success.

Appendices

Where are we at with the research?

It's hard to know if people are working to find a cure or at least better treatment options because no one is talking about it and what research *is* published is difficult to access or understand if you're not medically trained. I've spent hours online trying to make sense of complicated and distant documents written in abstract medical lingo so obscure that it's hard to remember they're discussing something which I'm actually experiencing. Because of this I've often felt 'forgotten' by science too; nothing seems to be changing. So on a freezing-cold but beautifully bright day, I went to the Endometriosis CaRe and Research Centre at Oxford University to speak to Professor Krina Zondervan, who is leading worldwide research into the disease. The clinic integrates clinical care (so they see patients), with cutting-edge, collaborative research.

E: Why does the current research focus on a genetic component?
K: Genetic research is being done on most diseases now, but for endometriosis it is particularly pertinent as there is a familial

component, though not for everyone. I think if we can understand the biology better, we can come up with more targeted treatments.

E: Is there a theory that there are different *types* of endometriosis?
K: Recent studies suggest that it is not one disease but probably multiple presentations of disease; ovarian disease might be quite different from peritoneal disease. So being able to identify sub-categories of disease will allow research programmes to really try and target those sub-types specifically.

E: Your work on biomarkers is ideally going to lead to a diagnostic test, like a blood test?
K: Yes, probably more of a screening test than a definite diagnosis. A screening test would, for example, mean that when a woman visits her GP with symptoms that may suggest endometriosis, the test can be done and she will know if there is a higher than average possibility that she has endometriosis. She can then be prioritised for referral to a specialist, rather than spending the current average of eight years trying to get a diagnosis.

E: Sounds great, how long till we get this?
K: A lot of companies are interested because of course there is money to be made from these kinds of screening tools. I think that with really solid funding backing, there's no reason why we shouldn't have something like this within five, maybe ten years. The potential is there, absolutely.

E: Someone once told me, rather frighteningly, that it's like a benign cancer in terms of how it grows?
K: So this is about the *features* of endometriosis. Endometriosis is basically a tissue that is in a place where it should not be, and that

is the same as any tumour, be it benign or malignant. That is one of the main characteristics of endometriosis, that you have endometrial tissue and cellular growth in places where that shouldn't occur. Another similarity with tumour formation is what we would call cellular invasion; cells that 'dig' into the peritoneum and grow, followed by the establishment of a blood supply, an invasion to essentially feed that bit of tissue there. All of these are hallmarks that you see in cancer, which are helpful to learn more about underlying biology. What makes endometriosis essentially *benign* is the fact that there is no metastasis, so there is no 'out of control' growth that impairs normal bodily functioning. In summary, although we think endometriosis has hallmarks of benign tumour formation and this is helpful for researching its biology, it is very important to emphasise that is where the similarity stops, and it is NOT cancer.

E: So it has similar growth patterns. Why does it help us to know that? Could it mean that in theory some treatments could be used to eradicate the disease for some women?

K: What is very interesting is that the discrimination between malignant versus benign is not just important from a health point of view, it's also relevant from a pharmaceutical point of view. In the cancer field there are lots of drug targets that are fairly acceptable as long as they are effective, they produce lots of side effects but ultimately they kill the tumour. But because endometriosis is a *benign disease*, and not lethal, the treatments would be too strong to use ethically, because they would just cause so many side effects that it would not be acceptable to a woman suffering from endometriosis. So we have to search hard for treatments that are acceptable, and do not make a woman with endometriosis feel worse than she already does.

E: Why is research collaboration important?
K: What we really need to focus on is taking a multi-disciplinary approach to research in endometriosis; basic research integrated with clinical studies involving women who have been diagnosed, and collaborations with industry so we can feed into their discovery programmes with novel ideas for new drugs. For instance, genetic research is not something that one centre can focus on alone, you need large collaborations, large studies. Therefore, we work together with many centres, currently up to 25 globally, to conduct genome studies.

So what have we learnt?
- Research so far indicates that early intervention, detection and specific treatment for the condition are the most urgent issues to address.
- We need to know more about the origins of disease, why and how it grows, in order to understand what to do to treat it and to manage it.
- Research is massively underfunded globally; this has to get better for anything to change in terms of treatments and diagnostic tools.
- There is a correlation between awareness of the condition and the impetus to invest more into the research of it. So until people truly know the effects on women's lives, the economy and the health system, there won't be the motivation to fund the research better.
- With more funding, research could lead to a development of specific drugs which would provide alternatives to surgical or hormonal management and less invasive diagnostic tests.
- Research is made more complicated because there isn't one

cohesive collection of data. This is partly down to funding but also because patients often see many doctors in different cities and countries, in different medical systems, some seek some help privately, or don't go back to the same doctor. But without a collective approach to this condition there can't be an overview of evidence that would help researchers make links, connections and see patterns.

* * *

Useful things all in one place

Where's my nearest endometriosis centre?
The BSGE (British Society for Gynaecological Endoscopy) lists the accredited centres in the UK here: https://www.bsge.org.uk/centre/

Understanding referrals and patient rights
Read more about the NICE (National Institute for Health and Care Excellence) guidelines on endometriosis here: https://www.nice.org.uk/guidance/ng73

For more support in appointments and navigating the medical system
Many NHS trusts have a PALS (Patient Advice and Liaison Service); enquire about this at your hospital or search online here: https://www.nhs.uk

Reliable, non-scary places to find info
Endometriosis UK: https://www.endometriosis-uk.org
This charity site also has links to local and online support groups near you.

Endometriosis Foundation of America: https://www.endofound.org

Other places for support
Adenomyosis Advice Association: https://www.adenomyosisadvice-association.org

Pelvic Pain Support Network: https://www.pelvicpain.org.uk

Hysterectomy Association: https://www.hysterectomy-association.org.uk

Forums:
https://myendometriosisteam.com
https://healthunlocked.com

Practical help
Pelvic Relief is a great company that sells items that can help with pelvic pain, incontinence and intimate health issues (such as painful sex). They have yoga blocks, lubricants, devices that help to relax and calm your body such as vibrators and dilators – which can help with over-sensitivity in the pelvic region https://www.pelvicrelief.co.uk

Mental-health support
Samaritans: https://www.samaritans.org
Mind: https://www.mind.org.uk

Employment-rights support:
ACAS (Advisory, Conciliation and Arbitration Service): www.acas.
org.uk

Some (other) helpful books:
Tamer Seckin MD, *The Doctor Will See You Now.* I loved this book;
he is clear, concise and hopeful. The most accessible medical book
I've found. I learnt stuff I didn't know even after twenty-three
years of having endometriosis. And it made me cry – in a good
way – to find someone who cares this much and who has dedicated their career to helping women suffering with this puzzling
disease.

Jill Eckersley and Dr Zara Aziz, *Coping with Endometriosis.*

Professor Andrew Horne and Carol Pearson, *Endometriosis: The
Experts' Guide to Treat, Manage and Live Well with Your Symptoms.*

Kerry-Ann Morris, *Living Well with Endometriosis: What Your Doctor
Doesn't Tell That You Need to Know.*

Dr Nina Brochmann and Dr Ellen Støkken Dahl, *The Wonder Down
Under.*

Dian Shepperson Mills MA and Michael Vernon PH HCLD,
Endometriosis: A Key to Healing and Fertility Through Nutrition.

Jessica Murnane, *One Part Plant.* Written by a fellow endometriosis
sufferer who uses diet to manage symptoms. The book is easy to
navigate, inspiring, but best of all, it's realistic because she knows
what it's like to try and tackle diet while living with endometriosis.

And now . . . some thanks

Zoe Ross and Gabriella Docherty at United Agents for huge support and guidance throughout. Judith Longman, Claire Hubbard, Melissa Cox, Lily Cooper, Vero Norton, Steven Cooper, Caitriona Horne, Susan Spratt and Sarah Christie at Hodder & Stoughton. Hannah Begbie, Maureen Vincent, Kitty Laing, Carly Peters and all at United Agents for your encouragement from the beginning. The Royal Society of Authors, for your enormous support, which helped me to get to the point where I can type this.

All the people who kindly advised on and were interviewed for the book: Mr Andrew Baxter, Mr Davor Jurkovic, Mr Michael Dooley, Professor Krina Zondervan, Ms Katy Vincent, Dr Jannie Van Der Merwe, Emma Cox CEO of Endometriosis UK, Mr Benjamin Rossi, Dr Emma Barnsley and Dr Tehseen Suleman.

Hilary Mantel for long talks and wheat-free cake. Lena Dunham for such kindness when I really needed it. Paulette Edwards for sharing your story so bigheartedly. Jessica Knappett for being there *always*, whether it's midnight hospital trips, performing in a show or a rude meal – always with love whatever and forever. Trevor Thompson for lifelong friendship, laughs, and inappropriate book titles. Tom Allen for late night calls, advice and huge friendship. Phoebe Waller-Bridge for your encouragement and kindness. Joe Lycett for offering to kick endometriosis in the dick and for being a true friend when it got dark. Will Wood for telling me this was a book and for always believing in me. Mick Perrin for your vision, patience and generosity. Jennifer Saunders for your love and company when I was at my sickest.

My family and friends, without whom I would be lost: Claire Benjamin, Emma Barnsley, Rose and John Redgrave, The Younies (Chris and Ben), Jess Barnett, Karl Gibbons, Hannah Marler (Lady Doddbeth), Alina Basu, Alice Storey, Jessica Gunning, Heather Jowitt, Diccon Ramsey, Sarah Thorniley-Walker, Dan Crane, Duckie Daniel Cooper, Alec Drysdale, Lucy Oliver-Harrison, Julia Charteris and Georgia Maguire. You never stopped the fun and brought it to me when I couldn't come to you. All the Robinsons, O'Sheas and Wasps for a lifetime of stories, songs and love.

Thanks to all the Chrises I have ever loved – you know who you are.

My brother Goronwy and sister Megan – I wouldn't have survived any of it without you. Rosie, Steph and Ben for guaranteed larks and laughs. Sandy, Flossie, Matilda, Ebon and Jolyon, you brighten my world. Pam Thom, for the pancakes and laughs. Sylvia Moorman for jaunts galore and for the enormous (and speedy) transcribing work. Viv Thom for teaching me to be brave and fierce, for helping me out of the bath, hot chickens, enduring love and of course *The West Wing* nights. Rony Robinson, the best writer I know, for unconditional love, support and belief, for magical mystery tours, for always being on the end of the phone to untangle words and life and for teaching me to find the laughs whenever you can.

Index